Pediatric Dyslipidemia

Ambika Ashraf • Bhuvana Sunil
Editors

Pediatric Dyslipidemia

A Practical Guide

Springer

Editors
Ambika Ashraf
Pediatrics
University of Alabama at Birmingham
Birmingham, AL, USA

Bhuvana Sunil
Department of Pediatrics
Mary Bridge Children's Hospital
Tacoma, WA, USA

ISBN 978-3-031-24112-3 ISBN 978-3-031-24113-0 (eBook)
https://doi.org/10.1007/978-3-031-24113-0

This Springer imprint is published by the registered company Springer Nature Switzerland AG
The registered company address is: Gewerbestrasse 11, 6330 Cham, Switzerland

Foreword

As the millennium progresses, clinical recognition of cardiovascular risk factors in children has become an increasingly important part of pediatric practice with not only the publication of evidence-based guidelines but also proven long-term success of treatments to lower cholesterol and to detect and manage acute and chronic hyperlipidemias. Nevertheless, translation to practice has been a challenge, partly because an assumed adult disease has not been fully recognized and understood by providers caring for children with demanding and multiproblem presentations. However, despite known barriers to detection and management, incorporation of informed information into practice has the potential to be resolved by presenting education on lipids in a usable format. This book achieves that goal leading to pediatric lipid abnormalities and their metabolic origins becoming solvable problems to serve patients and provide the best preventive practice leading to enduring cardiovascular health.

Of the key risk factors identified by pediatric expert committees, circulating lipids and lipoproteins have been prominent targets of interest, especially for cases with genetic disorders resulting in dyslipidemia beginning in infancy and therefore subjecting the child's vascular intima to lifelong exposures. Hypotheses that certain lipid particles in children lead to adverse cardiovascular outcomes have been further supported by Mendelian randomization studies comparing carriers of mutations with noncarriers and by follow-up data on long-term treatment studies. These outcomes signify an urgent call for better understanding and application in clinical settings.

Ambika Ashraf and Bhuvana Sunil have assembled a well-qualified team of experts to challenge pediatric lipid practice norms by reviewing the latest evidence as a basis for attaining excellence. The panel of expert authors have succeeded in presenting essential information for use in everyday practice. They have not only elucidated the origins of the particles containing cholesterol, triglyceride, phospholipid, and their key transporting proteins, but also provided insight on their circulation, disposal, and both their pathological and non-pathological destiny. The reader is also provided with ways to diagnose early disease and prevent progression based on new disease markers when indicated by unique clinical presentations, with insightful advice on the use of medications and lifestyle.

The first chapter begins with a historical account by Tanya Correya, Badhma Valiayapathi, and Ambika Ashraf who outline how pioneers in the field were inspired to investigate the cause of what then seemed an epidemic of fatal disease in adults. Basic investigation on lipid transport led to observation of derangements in lipid transport and to suspicion that disease began in childhood. Pioneers in pediatric lipidology were influenced by landmark pathological studies on youth and biochemical findings forming the basis for cohort studies from childhood to adulthood, and evidence-based guidelines on prevention and treatments.

Bhuvana Sunil and Ambika Ashraf continue with a chapter on the metabolism of cholesterol, illustrating how dramatic progress has led to understanding its origins and metabolic fate enabling the reader to conceptualize in three dimensions with a supportive diagram. Transitioning from theory to practice, Christy Foster, Bhuvana Sunil, and Ambika Ashraf outline guidelines for pediatric lipid screening according to evidence-based compilations by national expert panels. In Chap. 4, Marissa Lightbourne and Stephanie Chung, experts based at the National Institutes of Health, clarify why and how lipids and lipoproteins are measured, complementing the metabolic concepts presented in Chap. 2 and translating the biochemistry to use in practice. In Chap. 5, Adam Ware and Don Wilson, two prominent physician-scientist leaders in the field, provide a practical approach to low-density lipoprotein (LDL) disorders with case illustrations, a risk factor diagram and eight informative tables, and include information on management of low cholesterol disorders. Although relatively rare presentations, the disorders not only present as significant phenotypes with curable clinical manifestations but also provide valuable insight into the pathophysiological results of deficient nutrient transport. In Chap. 6, Nivedita Patni provides a masterful approach for LDL cholesterol lowering and includes the evidence base for adhering to national treatment guidelines with insight on mechanisms of action and adverse events including information on rare disorders.

There are examples of clinical presentations in both pediatric and adult practice where not all cases are the same, and with the right questions and careful study design, it becomes possible to subclassify providing frontline providers with insight on diagnosis, consideration of associated disease, and better treatment strategies based on an informed assessment. There is no better example of this than commonly encountered hypertriglyceridemia with a low HDL-C, and no better expert in the field than Rae-Ellen Kavey to clarify the topic of combined dyslipidemia (CD) and its strong association with multiple interrelated cardiometabolic risk factors. Since it often predominates as the presenting diagnosis in lipid clinic settings, management often takes center stage. In Chap. 8, Janet Carter, a highly qualified nutritionist, and Rae-Ellen Kavey present management of CD with emphasis on lifestyle and sensitivity to the demands of behavior change required for long-term success. Besides five supportive tables, each page of the chapter is packed with pearls of information.

Continuing with the theme and focus on triglyceride disorders, Chap. 9 is by Robert Hegele, a renowned Canadian geneticist and lipidologist who has had a long-standing interest in the genetics of hyperlipidemia contributing to its classification and scientific basis for treatments. The chapter provides information on mutations causing monogenic and multigenic forms of hypertriglyceridemia and focuses on severe familial chylomicronemia (FCS) with information on both conservative and new promising pharmacologic treatments.

Although discovered half a century ago, lipoprotein(a) has emerged as a significant risk factor worthy of study, accurate measurement, structure-function studies, and risk-specific guidelines on management including for at-risk children. Mostafa Salama and Seema Kumar have approached the topic based on the unique composition of its protein component, severity of its effects, and evidence-based pediatric guidelines. In the final chapter, Christy Foster, Bhuvana Sunil, and Ambika Ashraf discuss a collection of rare lipid and lipoprotein disorders, emphasizing a need for clinical recognition skills, challenge of correct diagnosis, and scientific breakthroughs leading to effective treatments.

Congratulations to the authors on their contributions not only for pediatric providers but also to all those concerned with the translation of lipid research and clinical experience to practice.

Endocrinology and Diabetes Section
Department of Pediatrics
University of Oklahoma Health Sciences Center
Oklahoma City, OK, USA

Piers R. Blackett

Preface

The vision behind this book, entitled **Pediatric Dyslipidemia: A Practical Guide**, was to create a comprehensive and easily accessible guide for quick referencing when lipid abnormalities are encountered in an office setting. The book is designed to include figures and tables with a clinical focus for accurate diagnosis and management of pediatric dyslipidemia. In addition, this book on pediatric dyslipidemia distinguishes itself by its concise nature, reader friendliness for trainees, practicing pediatricians, endocrinologists, and other subspecialists, emphasizing practical management strategies readily applicable in a busy clinical practice. Most of the chapters include clinical vignettes to discuss commonly encountered clinical scenarios. National and international leaders in pediatric lipidology contributed to the book, and we are grateful to the authors for their knowledge and invaluable contributions. We want to dedicate a special acknowledgment to children with dyslipidemia who taught us important lessons about primary prevention, risk mitigation, diagnosis, and management.

Birmingham, AL — Ambika Ashraf
Tacoma, WA — Bhuvana Sunil

Contents

Contributors

Ambika Ashraf Heersink School of Medicine, University of Alabama at Birmingham, Birmingham, AL, USA

Janet Carter Department of Pediatrics, Medical University of South Carolina/ Morrison Healthcare, Charleston, SC, USA

Stephanie T. Chung Diabetes, Endocrinology, and Obesity Branch, National Institute of Diabetes & Digestive & Kidney Diseases, National Institutes of Health, Bethesda, MD, USA

Tanya Correya Heersink School of Medicine, University of Alabama at Birmingham, Birmingham, AL, USA

Christy Foster Department of Pediatrics, University of Alabama at Birmingham, Birmingham, AL, USA

Robert A. Hegele Department of Medicine, Schulich School of Medicine and Dentistry, Western University, London, ON, Canada

Robarts Research Institute, Western University, London, ON, Canada

Rae-Ellen W. Kavey Department of Pediatrics, University of Rochester Medical Center, Rochester, NY, USA

Seema Kumar Division of Pediatric Endocrinology, Department of Pediatric and Adolescent Medicine, Mayo Clinic, Rochester, MN, USA

Marissa Lightbourne Diabetes, Endocrinology, and Obesity Branch, National Institute of Diabetes & Digestive & Kidney Diseases, National Institutes of Health, Bethesda, MD, USA

Nivedita Patni Department of Pediatrics, UT Southwestern Medical Center, Dallas, TX, USA

Mostafa Salama Division of Pediatric Endocrinology, Department of Pediatric and Adolescent Medicine, Mayo Clinic, Rochester, MN, USA

Bhuvana Sunil Department of Pediatric Endocrinology, Mary Bridge Children's Hospital, Tacoma, WA, USA

Badhma Valaiyapathi Department of Psychiatry-Behavioral Neurobiology, University of Alabama at Birmingham, Birmingham, AL, USA

Adam L. Ware Department of Pediatric Cardiology, University of Utah, Salt Lake City, UT, USA

Don P. Wilson Department of Pediatric Endocrinology and Diabetes, Cook Children's Medical Center, Fort Worth, TX, USA

Chapter 1
History and Significance of Pediatric Lipidology

Tanya Correya, Badhma Valaiyapathi, and Ambika Ashraf

Introduction

Lipidology, the scientific study of lipids is a relatively young field. Discovery of chylomicrons, triglycerides (TG), and lipoproteins allowed for a more nuanced understanding of the different types of lipids and lipoproteins, and their effects. Laboratory research, large-scale epidemiologic studies, Mendelian randomization studies, and clinical trials allowed to define cardiovascular disease (CVD) risk factors and novel therapeutic agents.

The field of lipidology started with identification of cholesterol, lipoproteins, and understanding their role in atherosclerosis. In 1910, Adolf Windaus proposed that atheromatous plaques are made of cholesterol. Subsequently, in 1919, cholesterol structure was described (A. O. Windaus) and in 1928, Windaus and Heinrich Wieland received the Nobel Prize for this work. In the late 1940s and 1950s, techniques to separate and quantify lipoprotein categories as very low (VLDL), low (LDL), and high (HDL) density lipoproteins were identified. In 1949–1950, John Gofman et al. from the University of California at Berkeley quantitatively measured

T. Correya
Heersink School of Medicine, University of Alabama at Birmingham, Birmingham, AL, USA
e-mail: tanya98@uab.edu

B. Valaiyapathi
Department of Psychiatry-Behavioral Neurobiology, University of Alabama at Birmingham, Birmingham, AL, USA
e-mail: bvalaiyapathi@uabmc.edu

A. Ashraf (✉)
Department of Pediatrics, University of Alabama at Birmingham, Birmingham, AL, USA
e-mail: aashraf@uabmc.edu

A. Ashraf, B. Sunil (eds.), *Pediatric Dyslipidemia*,
https://doi.org/10.1007/978-3-031-24113-0_1

serum lipoproteins using ultracentrifugation. In 1950, Ancel Keys formulated the cholesterol hypothesis postulating that hypercholesterolemia is related to CVD. Lipoprotein(a) [Lp(a)] was discovered in the 1960s by Kåre Berg in Norway.

The next major focus was prevention and management of CVD, which was identified as the number one cause of death in the United States by 1940. In 1947, Vartiainen reported that the incidence of atherosclerosis in Europe had declined during World War II and attributed this to changes in dietary intake. In 1948, President Harry Truman signed the National Heart Act, allocating $500,000 to fund the Framingham Heart Study and establish a National Heart Institute. The Framingham Study in adults was initiated by the National Heart Institute in 1948 to understand population risk and basis of CVD and is currently in its fourth generation of participants, providing decades of longitudinal analyses. The study would go on to enroll 5209 people in the original cohort with expansions to offspring, third generation, spouses of offspring, and more new diverse residents to the area [1]. Starting in the late 1950s, findings from the original cohort were published. Data obtained from this longitudinal study supports the role of diet and exercise in mitigating hypertension and arteriosclerotic CVD. In 1953, Enos et al. authored a paper describing evidence of coronary atherosclerosis found on 77.3% of the autopsies of 300 young-adult American soldiers killed in Korea, with an average age of 22 [2].

Dr. Donald Fredrickson's work paved the way for the creation of the study of lipidology. In 1965, Frederickson et al. published a classification system for phenotyping hyperlipidemia. He pioneered the work on cholesteryl ester storage diseases resulting from the deficiency of lysosomal enzyme activities. In 1972, Donald Fredrickson, William Friedewald, and Robert Levy created a convenient formula together for estimating LDL-C using the fasting lipid levels of TG, total cholesterol, and HDL-C. While the Friedewald-Levy-Fredrickson formula has its limitations, it provided an easy way to gauge LDL-C levels instead of using ultracentrifugation [3]. Subsequently by the 1990s, direct LDL-C measurements became possible.

In a continued effort to understand the population basis of CVD, the Muscatine Heart Study led by Dr. Ronald Lauer was the longest running study of CV risk factors in children in the United States. Six biennial school surveys were conducted between 1970 and 1981 with a total of 11,377 school children from Muscatine, Iowa undergoing 26,919 examinations that measured body size and risk factor levels.

The Bogalusa Heart Study was a long-term study on a rural biracial community initiated by Dr. Gerald Berenson in 1972 with NIH funding, as the population distribution of black/white was comparable to the southeast region of the United States [4]. Running for over 40 years, the epidemiological study followed 16,000 participants from birth to adulthood to determine heart disease incidence and risk factors. Dr. Gerald Berenson published "Cardiovascular Risk Factors in Children: The Early Natural History of Atherosclerosis and Essential Hypertension" in 1980 as his first book on the study.

Dr. Peter Kwiterovich was another pioneer in the field of pediatric lipidology. His extensive work helped establish normal cholesterol levels in children and how statin therapy can be safely administered to children with familial hypercholesterolemia.

He was the founder and director of the lipid clinic at Johns Hopkins. Along with Dr. Frederickson and Dr. Levy, Dr. Kwiterovich worked on neonatal diagnosis of familial type-II hyperlipoproteinemia in 1973.

In 1975, Dr. R Lowenthal, Dr. GR Thompson, and Dr. NB Myant studied the uses of plasma exchange in the management of homozygous familial hypercholesterolemia. Two young women with homozygous familial hypercholesterolemia participated in an outpatient plasma exchange treatment every 3 weeks for 4 and 8 months. The patients' angina disappeared, and they experienced significant decrease in plasma cholesterol and LDL-C.

In 1985, Dr. Michael Brown and Dr. Joseph Goldstein from the University of Texas received the Nobel Prize in Physiology or Medicine for their revolutionary discovery of the LDL receptor and its role in cholesterol metabolism.

Dr. Jack Strong was an internationally renowned pathologist who was a faculty member of the Louisiana Shreveport University Medical Center since 1955. He led the Pathobiological Determinants of Atherosclerosis in Youth (PDAY) Study in the United States, which is a comprehensive source regarding the origins of early heart disease in youth and its progression. He first established the link between smoking and heart disease.

In 1993, the importance of early recognition and treatment of heterozygous familial hypercholesterolemia (HeFH) for CVD prevention was illustrated by Roger Williams et al. based on a landmark study from the Utah Cardiovascular Genetics Research Clinic evaluating 502 patients with familial heterozygous familial hypercholesterolemia (HeFH). He showed that screening close family members of FH probands and subsequently identifying affected relatives was shown to be cost-effective approach, thus pioneering "cascade screening" leading to his development of an international initiative named MEDPED (Make an Early Diagnosis to Prevent Early Death). Incidentally, he died in a plane crash while travelling to a MEDPED meeting in 1998.

In 1995, Samuel Gidding et al. examined the pediatric population included in the Bogalusa Heart Study, a long-term epidemiologic study of cardiovascular risk factors in two biracial cohorts between 1973–1981 and 1984–1992. Comparison and secular trends showed that an overall weight gain of 2 kg occurred from the 1970s to the 1980s, and 5 kg from the 1980s to the 1990s and was associated with a more metabolic syndrome like pattern with low HDL-C and elevated TG levels [5]. Overall, risk factors including lipid panels, body mass index (BMI), blood pressure, and cigarette smoking were assessed. The study results published in 1998 demonstrated that with greater risk factors, a higher severity of asymptomatic coronary artery atherosclerosis was seen in children and young adults. Consequently, it was established that atherosclerosis began in childhood [6].

In 2000, the Pathobiological Determinants of Atherosclerosis in Youth (PDAY) Research Group led a study to look at atherosclerosis in adolescents and the risk for coronary artery disease. In this study, autopsies were done on 760 adolescents and young adults aged 15–34. Advanced atherosclerosis was found in 2% of 15–19-year-old men, 20% of 30–34-year-old men and 8% of 30–34-year-old women. This study demonstrated that young Americans have a high prevalence of coronary plaques and early prevention of hypercholesterolemia is critical in minimizing the risk of CVD [7].

The International Childhood Cardiovascular Cohort (i3C) consortium initiated in 2008 was the first study aiming to obtain longitudinal data linking childhood cardiovascular risk factors to adult cardiovascular disease. In 2008, Petar Alaupovic et al. published "Characterization of the metabolic syndrome by apolipoproteins in the Oklahoma Cherokee," based on the NIH-funded Oklahoma Cherokee Study on children and young adults from age 5 to 40 led by Elisa Lee.

The National Cholesterol Education Program (NCEP) was started in 1985, and published the first cholesterol guidelines NCEP Adult Treatment Panel (ATP 1) in 1988 which provided a strategy for preventing CHD in patients with high or borderline LDL-C levels of >160 mg/dL and 130–159 mg/dL, respectively. Lipid screening guidelines in pediatrics were first published in 1992. The panel comprised generalists and subspecialists to evaluate screening practices in children and adolescents. The report stated that children and adolescents have higher blood cholesterol and US adults have higher rates of CVD. Early coronary atherosclerosis or precursors had been identified by autopsy in children and adolescents. Elevated cholesterol was associated with early atherosclerotic lesions in young adulthood. In 1993, the second NCEP guidelines were published. The committee revised its initial guidelines with more of an emphasis on HDL-C levels, weight loss, and physical activity. Recommendations were made to add HDL-C to the initial cholesterol testing and designating high HDL-C as a negative risk factor for coronary heart disease. The second ATP guideline supported the approach of ATP-I and added a new feature of intensive management of LDL-C in patients with established CHD (secondary prevention) and fixed a new, lower LDL-C goal of <100 mg/dL in CHD patients. This recommendation is reinforced by clinical trials that show a reduction in morbidity and mortality of 30–50%.

In 2001, the NCEP released the *Third Report of the Expert Panel on Detection, Evaluation, and Treatment of High Blood Cholesterol in Adults, Adult Treatment Panel III* (ATP III) [8]. A modification of the Framingham risk scoring system was presented, with diabetes being considered a CHD equivalent, and risk factors were assigned for associations of age with smoking, age with total cholesterol, and systolic blood pressure with treatment. In 2004, NCEP ATP III was updated when landmark statin trials were completed.

In the pediatric realm, in 2011, NHLBI guidelines were published for management of pediatric dyslipidemia. These guidelines were mostly in line with the NCEP and suggested no routine lipid screening before age 8 years. In children 2–8 years of age, higher risk selective screening was recommended. Universal screening was recommended for low-risk individuals at age 9–11 years and 17–21 years. These recommendations for universal screening, while controversial at the time, recognized LDL-C levels as a contributor to heart disease, and outlined primary prevention strategies [9]. It emphasized that non-fasting total cholesterol and non-high-density lipoprotein cholesterol (non-HDL-C) could be used for the initial lipid screening test. The goal was to recognize familial hypercholesterolemia (FH), with a high prevalence of one in 300–500 children but clinically silent until there was ASCVD. It outlined dietary management for nearly everyone for up to 6 months, and pharmacotherapy for selected individuals with higher risk of obvious FH. It provided an algorithmic integration of high- and moderate level risk factors and conditions, a helpful framework for setting targets to start therapy, and involved monitoring and therapeutic goals.

In 2010, The Cardiac Project led by William Neal in the West Virginia Appalachians resulted in a publication by Richie et al. on "Universal versus targeted blood cholesterol screening among youth: The CARDIAC project" investigating the role of family history to identify children with genetic or severe dyslipidemia. A National Heart Lung and Blood Institute (NHLBI) expert Panel lead by Stephen Daniels formulated an updated guidelines for cardiovascular health and risk reduction in youth in 2011. The American Heart Association outlined further management of pediatric dyslipidemia in children and provided specific high-risk related guidelines in 2019 [10].

Lipid Lowering Medications

While scientists were discovering the novel mechanisms of the role of cholesterol in diseases, pharmacotherapeutics were being developed for the optimal treatment of lipid disorders. In 1955, niacin became the first agent shown to reduce cholesterol levels. In 1959, cholestyramine was the first bile sequestrant shown to reduce cholesterol levels and was the first bile acid sequestrant (BAS), to be approved by the FDA in 1973. Two years later, fenofibrate, a drug mainly used to lower TG, first became available for medical use and was subsequently approved by the FDA in 1993. In 1981, the FDA approved gemfibrozil, a drug used for very high blood levels of TG to lower pancreatitis risk and increase HDL-C.

In 1987, lovastatin was the first statin approved for decreasing hepatic cholesterol synthesis through HMG CoA reductase inhibition. Since then, 7 more statins were studied and approved including pravastatin, atorvastatin, fluvastatin, cerivastatin, simvastatin, pitavastatin, and rosuvastatin. In 1991, pravastatin was the first statin approved for children 8 years of age and older with HeFH after failing a trial of dietary changes. The pediatric population studies in 2003 have shown pravastatin decreases LDL-C by 39% from baseline after 26 weeks [11]. Of the statins, rosuvastatin was one of the later ones to be approved in 2003 [12, 13]. In 2012, the FDA announced a small increased risk of type 2 diabetes, memory loss, and confusion in adults but said that evidence revealed that the risk was small. The need to monitor liver enzymes with statin use was also lifted by the FDA considering the evidence that this was overall exceedingly rare. In 2017, a large meta-analysis with over 130,000 studied participants showed its overall favorable side effect profile [14]. A 20-year follow-up from pediatric patients is now available showing that initiation of statin therapy during childhood in patients with FH slowed the atherosclerotic progression and reduced the risk of cardiovascular disease in adulthood [15].

Ezetimibe was approved for medical use in the United States in 2002. The ezetimibe/simvastatin combination pill was approved in 2004 for adults, and ezetimibe/rosuvastatin in 2021. In 2007, ezetimibe was approved for pediatric use when co-administered daily with approved doses of a statin for the treatment of HeFH. Ezetimibe 10 mg/day is approved by the FDA for use in children aged 10 and older.

In 2018, publication of REDUCE-IT provided the first proof of CVD reduction with a prescription omega-3 (icosapent-ethyl), and with any TG-lowering agent, when added to full-dose statin therapy. Mipomersen was not approved by the European Medicines Agency (EMA) in 2013 due to safety concerns from cardiovascular and hepatic adverse reactions. FDA approval for adults has since been discontinued.

The past two decades have witnessed a remarkable transition in research from bench to bedside with proprotein convertase subtilisin/kexin type 9 (PCSK9, an enzyme which catabolizes the LDL receptor) inhibitors. By the 2000s, *LDLR* and *APOB* were recognized genetic mutations leading to autosomal dominant hypercholesterolemia (ADH). Excess PCSK9 protein was discovered as a novel cause of FH in 2003, which led to initiating the development of PCSK9 inhibitors. There are increasing pediatric data for use of PCSK9 inhibitors. The HAUSER-RCT study, a 24-week double-blind, randomized controlled trial was conducted to evaluate the efficacy and safety of evolocumab treatment in pediatric patients with HeFH. The TAUSSIG study, an open-label, single-arm, multicenter study was conducted to evaluate the efficacy and safety of evolocumab in the long-term treatment of adults and adolescents with HoFH or severe HeFH ≥12 years of age. The study included 14 patients with HoFH <18 years of age at enrollment.

Data from the TESLA Part B trial in 2015 and the TAUSSIG study contributed towards the approval of evolocumab in combination with diet and other LDL-C lowering therapies in children ≥12 years. The HAUSER-RCT study included 157 children with HeFH and showed significant LDL-C reduction in addition to good drug tolerability. The ODYSSEY KIDS study assessed the efficacy and safety of alirocumab in HeFH. More clinical trials are underway that are further supportive of the use of these medications in children with HoFH (NCT03510715) and HeFH (NCT03510884). Evolocumab 420 mg by subcutaneous injection once monthly is approved for HeFH patients 10 years of age and older as adjunctive therapy.

In 2020, bempedoic acid, the first ATP citrate lyase inhibitor, was approved for lowering cholesterol in adults with HeFH or a prior CVD event. The following year in 2021, evinacumab was the first ANGPTL3 inhibitor approved for cholesterol lowering in adults with HoFH. Several pediatric trials are underway for the use of newer lipid-lowering medications targeting LDL-C and TG at the time of writing this chapter.

Even though the field of lipidology rapidly developed in the late twentieth century, with studies primarily focusing on FH and the development of lipid disorders as early as childhood, there were only a few clinics dedicated towards pediatric lipidology. As late as the 1990s, there were only three pediatric lipid clinics in the

Unites States which increased to 25 as of 2017. The disturbingly high prevalence of dyslipidemia in youth created a heightened awareness of new opportunities and challenges for pediatric endocrinologists. In 2019, Drs. Ambika Ashraf and Brenda Kohn established the Lipid Special Interest Group (SIG) within the Pediatric Endocrinology Society. The National Lipid Association has a Pediatric Atherosclerosis Prevention and Lipidology (PeDAL) Group with the purpose of advancing the field through research and education. Lipidology as a clinical discipline under pediatric endocrinology has evolved remarkably over the last decade.

Conclusion

This chapter has focused on the evolution of pediatric lipidology over the years. Clinical research on lipid-lowering agents has advanced rapidly and remarkably in the last two decades.

References

1. Mahmood SS, et al. The Framingham heart study and the epidemiology of cardiovascular disease: a historical perspective. Lancet. 2014;383(9921):999–1008.
2. Enos WF, Holmes RH, Beyer J. Coronary disease among United States soldiers killed in action in Korea; preliminary report. J Am Med Assoc. 1953;152(12):1090–3.
3. Friedewald WT, Levy RI, Fredrickson DS. Estimation of the concentration of low-density lipoprotein cholesterol in plasma, without use of the preparative ultracentrifuge. Clin Chem. 1972;18(6):499–502.
4. Berenson GS, Bogalusa Heart Study Investigators. Bogalusa heart study: a long-term community study of a rural biracial (black/white) population. Am J Med Sci. 2001;322(5):293–300.
5. Gidding SS, et al. Effects of secular trends in obesity on coronary risk factors in children: the Bogalusa heart study. J Pediatr. 1995;127(6):868–74.
6. Berenson GS, et al. Association between multiple cardiovascular risk factors and atherosclerosis in children and young adults. The Bogalusa heart study. N Engl J Med. 1998;338(23):1650–6.
7. McGill HC Jr, et al. Association of Coronary Heart Disease Risk Factors with microscopic qualities of coronary atherosclerosis in youth. Circulation. 2000;102(4):374–9.
8. Expert Panel on Detection, Evaluation, and Treatment of High Blood Cholesterol in Adults. Executive summary of the third report of the National Cholesterol Education Program (NCEP) Expert panel on detection, evaluation, and treatment of high blood cholesterol in adults (adult treatment panel III). JAMA. 2001;285(19):2486–97.
9. Expert Panel on Integrated Guidelines for Cardiovascular Health and Risk Reduction in Children and Adolescents, National Heart, Lung, and Blood Institute. Expert panel on integrated guidelines for cardiovascular health and risk reduction in children and adolescents: summary report. Pediatrics. 2011;128(Suppl 5):S213.
10. De Ferranti SD, et al. Cardiovascular risk reduction in high-risk pediatric patients: a scientific statement from the American Heart Association. Circulation. 2019;139(13):e603–34.
11. McCrindle BW, Ose L, Marais AD. Efficacy and safety of atorvastatin in children and adolescents with familial hypercholesterolemia or severe hyperlipidemia: a multicenter, randomized, placebo-controlled trial. J Pediatr. 2003;143(1):74–80.

12. Food and Drug Administration. Drugs@ FDA: FDA approved drug products. 2016.
13. Rosenson RS. Rosuvastatin: a new inhibitor of HMG-coA reductase for the treatment of dyslipidemia. Expert Rev Cardiovasc Ther. 2003;1(4):495–505.
14. Riaz H, et al. Meta-analysis of placebo-controlled randomized controlled trials on the prevalence of statin intolerance. Am J Cardiol. 2017;120(5):774–81.
15. Luirink IK, et al. 20-year follow-up of statins in children with familial hypercholesterolemia. N Engl J Med. 2019;381:1547.

Chapter 2
An Overview of Lipid Metabolism

Bhuvana Sunil and Ambika Ashraf

Introduction

Cholesterol and triglyceride form the two main lipids in the body. Lipoproteins are proteins that bind and transport lipids to its various target tissues. The lipoprotein comprises esterified and unesterified cholesterol, triglycerides (TG), phospholipids, and proteins.

Understanding Simple and Complex Lipids

Fatty acids, the building blocks of lipids are identified by the number of carbon atoms and the position of the double bond. ω-3 fatty acids like eicosapentaenoic (EPA) and docosahexaenoic (DHA) and ω-6 fatty acids like linoleic and arachidonic acid are considered essential as these cannot be endogenously synthesized. A *triglyceride* (TG) contains three stearic acid molecules connected to glycerol by ester linkages. A *lipoprotein* contains a core of TG and cholesterol surrounded by phospholipids.

B. Sunil (✉)
Department of Pediatric Endocrinology, Mary Bridge Children's Hospital, Tacoma, WA, USA

A. Ashraf
Department of Pediatrics, University of Alabama at Birmingham, Birmingham, AL, USA
e-mail: aashraf@uabmc.edu

A. Ashraf, B. Sunil (eds.), *Pediatric Dyslipidemia*,
https://doi.org/10.1007/978-3-031-24113-0_2

Exogenous Pathway of Lipid Metabolism

This starts with the intestinal absorption of cholesterol and fatty acids. Simple sugars and fructose substantially contribute towards TG synthesis. Dietary TG are hydrolyzed to release FFA by intestinal lipases, emulsified with cholesterol and bile acids and when available, plant sterols and fat-soluble vitamins to form micelles, facilitated by a sterol transporter, Niemann-Pick C1- like 1 protein (NPC1L1) [1]. Cholesterol and plant sterols are transported into the intestinal lumen by ABCG5 and ABCG8 [2]. Acyl-CoA cholesterol acyl transferase (ACAT) attaches a fatty acid to the sterol and esterifies these absorbed sterols [3]. FFA are transported by passive diffusion and via specific transporters like CD36.

Dietary TGs and cholesterol are assembled intracellularly as chylomicrons for which apoB48 is the main apolipoprotein. ApoCII is acquired during absorption. These are transported into the bloodstream through the thoracic duct, where they bind to the endothelium and are hydrolyzed by the action of lipoprotein lipase. Of the cofactors that are important in this pathway, apoCII activates upon LPL, promotes hydrolysis of the TG, and makes the core TG smaller, while releasing free fatty acids (FFA) in the process. ApoCIII, Angiopoietin-like 3 (ANGPTL3) and ANGPTL4 are known to inhibit the process of hydrolysis [4]. The released FFA can be taken up by adipose tissue to form TG again, or into the muscles for utilization. The chylomicron remnants that include intermediate density lipoprotein (IDL), very-low density lipoprotein (VLDL), TG-rich lipoproteins (TRLP) and lipoprotein(a) are cleared by the liver. ApoE serves as a highly selective ligand to aid this clearance process [4]. In the liver, these remnants can be used to synthesize HDL in the right metabolic milieu. After hydrolysis of the TG core, the resultant remnant chylomicron is high in cholesterol esters highlighted by apoproteins B, CIII, and E. When endocytosed into hepatocytes, they are catabolized by lysosomes liberating cholesterol, which is then converted into bile acids and excreted in bile—some of which are reabsorbed or incorporated into VLDL [4]. Figure 2.1 represents an overview of the exogenous cholesterol metabolism.

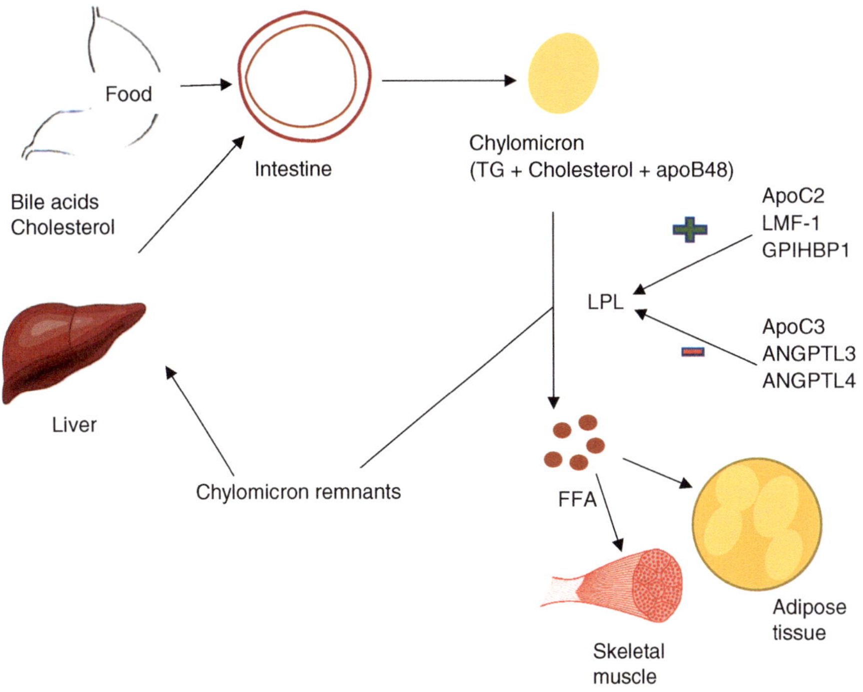

Fig. 2.1 Exogenous cholesterol metabolism pathway. Hydrolysis by the action of LPL releases FFA, chylomicron remnants, VLDL remnants, and intermediate density lipoproteins. Inhibition of LPL causes chylomicronemia and elevated TG, TRLP, and VLDL levels. *TG* triglyceride, *LPL* lipoprotein, lipase, *ANGPTL 3 and 4* angiopoietin-like proteins 3 and 4, *FFA* free fatty acid, *GPIHBP1* glycosylphosphatidylinositol-anchored high-density lipoprotein binding protein-1, *ABCA1* ATP Binding Cassette Subfamily A Member 1, *HL* hepatic lipase, *APOC2* apolipoprotein C2, *LMF-1* lipase maturation factor 1, *APOC3* apolipoprotein C3, *TRLP* triglyceride-rich lipoprotein, *LPL* lipoprotein lipase

Endogenous Pathway of Lipid Metabolism

VLDL particles, which contain about 60% cholesterol by mass are secreted from the liver. Hepatocytes synthesize VLDL by packaging TG and cholesterol with phospholipids and apo B100 by using FFAs and simple sugars as substrates in the presence of the microsomal triglyceride transfer protein (MTP), which facilitates the transfer of apoB to VLDL. The surface of VLDL has apo C-II (cofactor for LPL); apoC-III (LPL inhibitor); and apoB and apoE. In the capillary lumen, with the permissive action of GPIHBP1 (glycosylphosphatidylinositol-anchored high-density lipoprotein binding protein 1), VLDL is hydrolyzed by LPL, generating IDL, LDL and nascent HDL, each of which have more cholesterol content than their predecessor. In addition to hydrolysis, LPL also facilitates transfer of the apolipoproteins during this process [5]. As in the endogenous pathway, the FFA released during the process of hydrolysis are utilized in the skeletal muscle or stored in the adipose tissue. VLDL remnants can either be cleared from the circulation by LDL-R on the surface of hepatocytes which intake LDL or remodeled by hepatic lipase to form LDL particles which in turn are taken up by the LDL-R. Liver X receptors (LXRs) and farnesoid X receptor (FXR) are nuclear receptors working as sensors for sterols and bile acids and regulate cholesterol and bile acid metabolism. LXRs facilitate storage of carbohydrate- and fat-derived energy, whereas FXR activation results in an overall decrease in TG levels and modulation of glucose metabolism [5]. Figure 2.2 provides an overview of the exogenous cholesterol pathway.

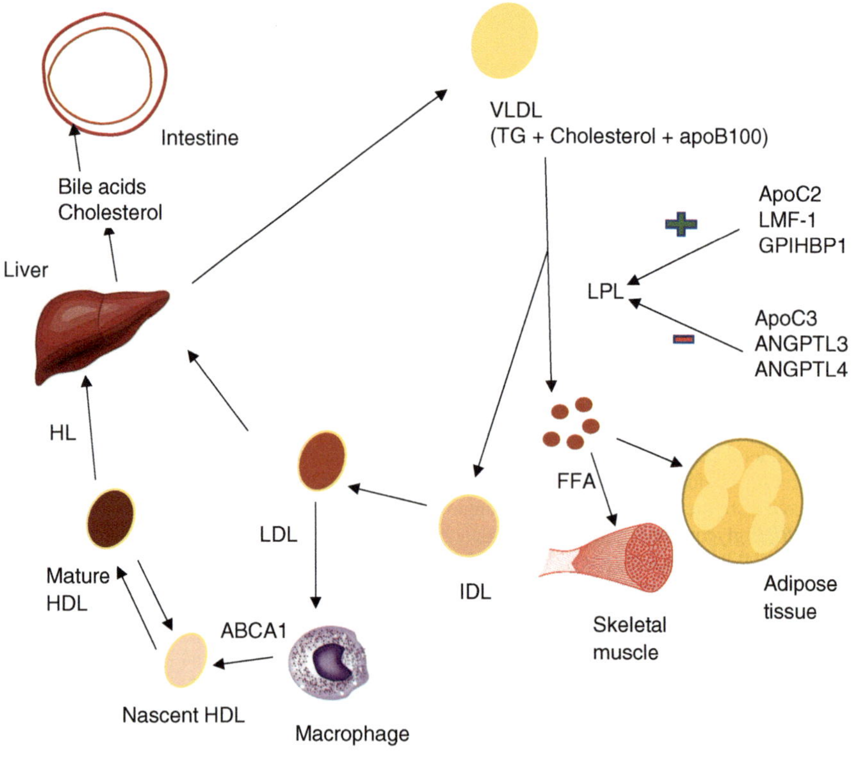

Fig. 2.2 Exogenous cholesterol metabolism pathway. Hydrolysis of the secreted VLDL by the action of LPL releases FFA, chylomicron remnants, IDL and eventually, LDL. The released FFA can be stored or utilized. LDL when oxidized by macrophages can eventually lead to the formation of foam cells and premature atherosclerosis. Nascent HDL facilitates some reverse cholesterol transport by transporting cholesterol back to the liver. LDL is taken up by the hepatocytes with the LDL-R. *TG* triglyceride, *LPL* lipoprotein, lipase, *ANGPTL 3 and 4* angiopoietin-like proteins 3 and 4, *FFA* free fatty acid, *GPIHBP1* glycosylphosphatidylinositol-anchored high-density lipoprotein binding protein-1, *IDL* intermediate density lipoprotein, *LDL* low-density lipoprotein, *HDL* high-density lipoprotein, *ABCA1* ATP Binding Cassette Subfamily A Member 1, *HL* hepatic lipase, *APOC2* apolipoprotein C2, *LMF-1* lipase maturation factor 1, *APOC3* apolipoprotein C3, *LPL* lipoprotein lipase

LDL, once taken up can be used for the synthesis of bile acids—which are then excreted into bile. Some of these undergo recycling through the enterohepatic circulation, while a portion is excreted in the stools. HMG Co A reductase is the rate-limiting step that controls de novo cholesterol synthesis—when downregulated, it can lead to increased expression of LDL-R and LDL uptake by the liver [5].

Reverse Cholesterol Transport

In the endogenous pathway, the generated nascent HDL particles promote the uptake and transfer of cholesterol by forming mature HDL through the action of ATP Binding Cassette Subfamily A Member 1 (ABCA1). Lecithin:cholesterol acyl transferase (LCAT) is the enzyme responsible for esterification of the HDL after it has acquired cholesterol. The cholesteryl ester transfer protein (CETP) transfers cholesteryl esters from HDL to TRLPs, LDL, and VLDL [6]. In this process, HDL-cholesterol is decreased, cholesterol in VLDL is increased, and LDL becomes smaller and denser. Intracellular CETP in both the periphery and the liver promote hepatic uptake and peripheral utilization [6].

LDL and Atherosclerosis

Landmark studies have shown that the atherosclerotic process begins in childhood and provides a strong association between LDL, apoB, and premature progressive atherosclerosis [7, 8]. ApoB is the predominant apolipoprotein for LDL and in general, measurement of apoB is a good indicator of all the atherogenic cholesterol particles in the body. Circulating LDL not taken up by LDL-R can be scavenged by macrophages and oxidized, which in turn chemoattract monocytes and promote conversion to macrophages and can also directly promote endothelial damage. These foam cells, in a pro-inflammatory milieu upregulate endothelial adhesiveness. When foam cells rupture, oxidized LDL is released, intracellular enzymes are activated, and oxygen-free radicals are released that further damage the vessel wall. They cause an increase in platelet aggregation, vasoconstriction, and intravascular thrombus formation [9].

Conclusions

Plasma cholesterol concentrations are dependent on the balance between synthesis through the endogenous pathway and absorption of dietary and biliary cholesterol through the exogenous pathway. The liver has a central role for cholesterol production and homoeostasis. Environmental factors and metabolic disturbances such as diabetes and obesity as well as genetic factors influence the level of cholesterol in blood, influencing inflammation and endothelial function promoting LDL uptake and accelerating plaque formation. Knowledge of the pathways can help understand and explore therapeutic targets for cholesterol lowering.

References

1. Altmann SW, et al. Niemann-pick C1 like 1 protein is critical for intestinal cholesterol absorption. Science. 2004;303(5661):1201–4.
2. Yu L, et al. Overexpression of ABCG5 and ABCG8 promotes biliary cholesterol secretion and reduces fractional absorption of dietary cholesterol. J Clin Invest. 2002;110(5):671–80.
3. Chang TY, et al. Acyl-coenzyme a: cholesterol acyltransferases. Am J Physiol Endocrinol Metab. 2009;297(1):E1–9.
4. Shepherd J. The role of the exogenous pathway in hypercholesterolaemia. Eur Heart J Suppl. 2001;3(suppl_E):E2–5.
5. Feingold KR, Grunfeld C. Introduction to lipids and lipoproteins. In: Endotext. South Dartmouth (MA): MDText.com, Inc., 2015.
6. Tall A. An overview of reverse cholesterol transport. Eur Heart J. 1998;19:A31–5.
7. McGill HC Jr, McMahan CA. Determinants of atherosclerosis in the young. Pathobiological determinants of atherosclerosis in youth (PDAY) research group. Am J Cardiol. 1998;82(10):30T–6T.
8. Berenson GS, et al. Association between multiple cardiovascular risk factors and atherosclerosis in children and young adults. N Engl J Med. 1998;338(23):1650–6.
9. Steinbrecher UP, Zhang H, Lougheed M. Role of oxidatively modified LDL in atherosclerosis. Free Radic Biol Med. 1990;9(2):155–68.

Chapter 3
Lipid Screening in for Pediatrics

Christy Foster, Bhuvana Sunil, and Ambika Ashraf

Rationale for Screening

Children with dyslipidemia are at risk for developing early atherosclerosis-related premature cardiovascular disease (CVD) or strokes as adults. Children with familial hypercholesterolemia (FH) (prevalence 1 in 300) and familial combined hyperlipidemia (FCH) (prevalence 1 in 100) experience lifelong cumulative exposure to elevated low-density cholesterol levels (LDL-C) and a projected 20% increase in risk for premature CVD [1]. The absence of physical stigmata characteristic of hypercholesterolemia (i.e., xanthoma and xanthelasma) in childhood makes it difficult to identify this at-risk population without universal screening. With the increasing incidence of obesity, insulin resistance, metabolic syndrome, prediabetes and type 2 diabetes, non-genetic causes of dyslipidemia are manifested at younger ages and exacerbated in severity. Use of family history may be inaccurate due to variability of definitions or unreliable and/or unavailable family history. A positive family history is absent in as many as 30–60% of those with elevated cholesterol. Similarly, family members may have been undiagnosed and unscreened. Screening non-fasting serum lipid profiles are good initial tests for children with dyslipidemia to identify high-risk individuals. Half of children and adolescents with dyslipidemia continue to have dyslipidemia as adults. Although large trials demonstrating the effectiveness of screening in all children are lacking, evidence for universal screening comes from demonstrating the high prevalence of FH and FCH, effectiveness of prevention in

C. Foster (✉) · A. Ashraf
Department of Pediatrics, University of Alabama at Birmingham, Birmingham, AL, USA
e-mail: cafoster@uabmc.edu; aashraf@uabmc.edu

B. Sunil
Department of Pediatric Endocrinology, Mary Bridge Children's Hospital, Tacoma, WA, USA
e-mail: Bhuvana.sunil@multicare.org

A. Ashraf, B. Sunil (eds.), *Pediatric Dyslipidemia*,
https://doi.org/10.1007/978-3-031-24113-0_3

these high-risk children, and studies demonstrating that atherosclerosis begins in childhood. Prior studies have shown that early identification of risk factors and timely interventions can result in improvement in total cholesterol (TC) and LDL-C. The harms of detection and early screening include labeling children whose lipid abnormalities may not persist into adulthood. There is also lack of data on cost-effectiveness data and concerns for multiple repeated lipid panels, downstream testing or the resultant anxiety in children with borderline lipid dysfunction.

Lipid Screening Recommendations

In 2011, the National Heart, Lung, and Blood Institute (NHLBI) recommended "universal screening" for 9–11-year-old children with a non-fasting lipid panel and if normal, a repeat lipid panel at age 17–21 years. The lipid panel should include direct measurement of TC, high density lipoprotein cholesterol (HDL-C), and triglycerides (TG). LDL-C can be derived using the Friedewald formula or the Martin-Hopkins modification and is fairly accurate unless the TG >400 mg/dL. In the case of an abnormal lipid profile (i.e., non-HDL-C >145 mg/dL, HDL-C <40 mg/dL, LDL-C >130 mg/dL, TG >100 mg/dL if child ≤10 years of age or TG >130 mg/dL if >10 years of age), repeating a fasting a lipid profile between 2 weeks and 3 months of the initial lipid panel is recommended. The values are then averaged to make further recommendations.

Children with risk factors or conditions (Fig. 5.1) will require a fasting lipid profile (targeted/selective screening) between ages 2–8 and 12–16 years [2]. The NHLBI has defined several risk factors and conditions in children. The recent AHA guidelines modified the nomenclature as "at risk, moderate risk and high risk" categories [3]. The selective/targeted screening is also recommended for children ages 2–8 years old as well as 12–16 years old if they have first or second degree relatives with a history of CVD or history of total cholesterol >240 mg/dL (Fig. 3.1).

Both LDL-C and non-HDL-C are used as targets to evaluate the CVD-related risks associated with dyslipidemia. It is important to note that calculation of non-HDL-C can be done when using a non-fasting sample. Non-HDL-C is calculated as the difference between total cholesterol and HDL-C [4]. The Bogalusa heart study has proven that non-HDL-C is a sensitive screening for dyslipidemia [5]. A non-fasting lipid profile is therefore excellent for screening as the non-HDL-C calculations are unaffected by hypertriglyceridemia. This is an attractive option since it provides an opportunity to screen at the time of the clinic visit without fasting. There are no clinical tools widely available to assess the progression of atherosclerosis in children currently.

Lipid screening guidelines by the NHLBI is endorsed by several professional societies, including the American Academy of Pediatrics (AAP), American Heart Association (AHA), and National Lipid Association (NLA). The 2008 National Institute for Health and Care Excellence guidelines and the 2015 consensus statement of the European Atherosclerosis Society recommend selective screening and cascade screening to identify children and adults with familial hypercholesterolemia.

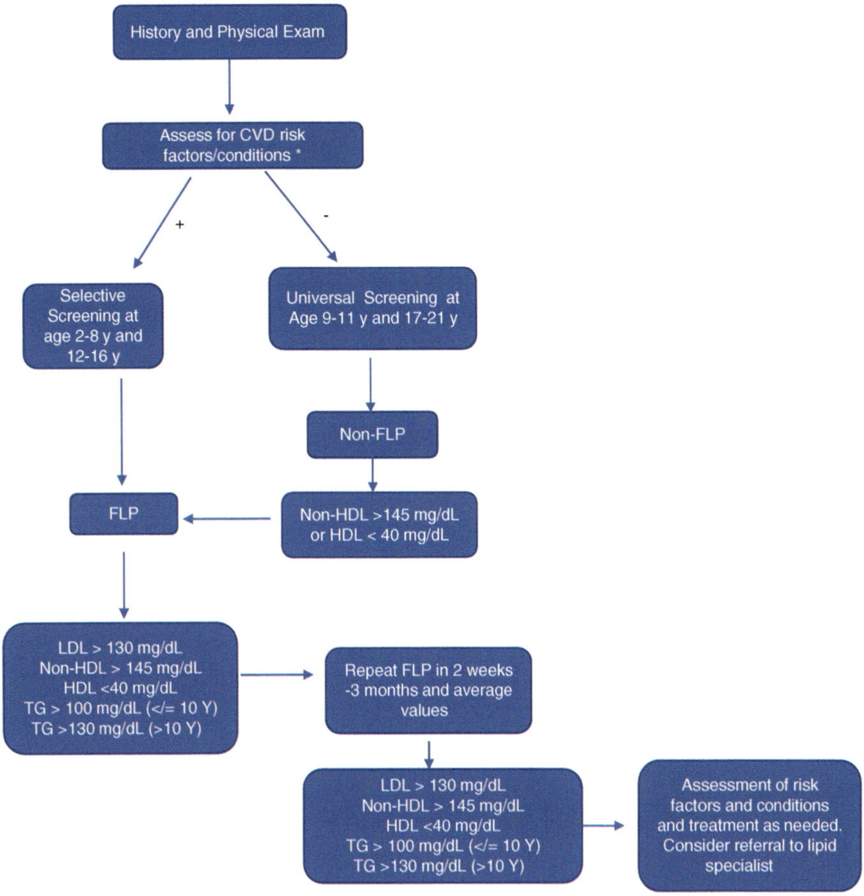

Fig. 3.1 Algorithm for Screening for Dyslipidemia in Children and Adolescents. *FLP* fasting lipid profile, *LDL* low-density lipoprotein, *HDL* high-density lipoprotein, *TG* triglycerides *Y* year. ASCVD risk factors: Positive family history of hypercholesterolemia or premature cardiovascular disease, high-risk conditions including Kawasaki disease, type 1 or type 2 diabetes, HIV or a solid organ transplant or nephrotic syndrome

The US Preventive Services Task Force (USPSTF) felt there was insufficient evidence to support the consistent screening for pediatric dyslipidemia.

All patients identified with dyslipidemia should have heart healthy lifestyle modification counseling. The NHBLI recommends continuing to reassess risk factors at each visit and to assess for secondary causes including hypothyroidism, diabetes, chronic liver, and/or kidney disease, use of medications such as steroids that may alter the lipid profile. For borderline abnormal values (i.e., between the 75th and 95th percentile—see below), repeat screening is suggested every 1–2 years. Decisions regarding medication therapy should be made on an individual basis.

Cascade Screening

Cascade screening is a mechanism for identifying people at risk for FH: Once an index patient with FH is identified, it is suggested to perform cascade screening of the first-degree relatives (i.e., parents, siblings, children). If an affected parent is identified, as many relatives as possible on that parent's side of the family should be screened. This screening involves identifying those first-, second-, and third-degree relatives of a patient with FH [6]. Each new case found via cascade screening then becomes a proband for broader cascading. The Centers for Disease Control and Prevention recommends cascade screening for FH based on systematic reviews that support integration into clinical and public health programs.

The indication for genetic testing is controversial, i.e., genetic testing is not necessary for a diagnosis of heterozygous FH as the treatment guidelines are based on LDL-C levels, rather than the specific genetic defect. Moreover, the genetic testing does not appear to predict responsiveness to statin therapy (except in case of homozygous FH), and several patients with clinical lipid phenotype for FH may have negative genetic testing.

Reference Ranges of Lipid Values by Age

Serum lipid values can vary by age through childhood and can be impacted by gender, race, and other factors as illustrated by the National Health and Nutrition Examination Survey from 1988–1994 and the National Health and Nutrition Survey from 1999–2006. Based on this the percentile curves were constructed, and normative values were defined [7]. In the Cardiovascular Health in Children Study of 8–10-year-olds in North Carolina, black children had the highest prevalence of having a total serum cholesterol concentration of >200 mg/dL: 18.7%, compared with 11% in white children [5]. Females tend to have higher TC and LDL-C compared to males. Females also had higher HDL-C levels as well compared to males. Black children had higher HDL-C compared to non-Hispanic white and Hispanic children [7].

The NCEP pediatric report from 1992 presented cut-off points to be used to identify children and adolescents with abnormal lipid and lipoprotein concentrations [8]. TC concentration peaks at ~170 mg/dL at 9–11 years of age. The values will then decrease during pubertal development—these changes in lipids decrease the sensitivity and specificity of screening during pubertal progression. In the absence of risk factors, routine screening between 12 and 16 years of age is not recommended for this reason. After 18 years of age, the adult lipid reference intervals should be utilized [8].

References specific for pediatric patients were released in the 2011 NHLBI expert guidelines (see Table 5.1)

Epidemiology

In the United States, approximately 20 percent of children between ages 6 and 19 years have abnormal lipid profiles. There were approximately 7.1% of those with elevated total cholesterol, 6.4% of children with elevated LDL-C, and 10.2% of children with elevated triglycerides. Longitudinal studies suggest that elevated LDL-C levels in adolescents predict elevated LDL-C 15–20 years later. FH is an autosomal dominant condition secondary to a mutation affecting the function of the LDL receptor. FCH is also a condition secondary to delayed clearance of triglyceride-rich lipoproteins with a prevalence of 1: 100. Individuals with this condition tend to have an increased risk of cardiovascular events, such as premature cardiovascular disease and strokes [9].

In the United States, in adolescents age 12–19, the prevalence of hypertriglyceridemia is approximately 10% [10]. Often, it appears secondary to underlying conditions including obesity, insulin resistance, type 1 diabetes, type 2 diabetes, renal or liver disease. The major causes of genetic hypertriglyceridemia include lipoprotein lipase (LPL) deficiency, which has an incidence of 1 in 500,000, and dysbetalipoproteinemia, which has an incidence of 1 in 5000 [10]. Cases with intermediate levels are often found to be multigenic and susceptible to exacerbation by secondary causes (see Chap. 9).

Clinical Case

A 10-year-old boy presented for a well-child visit. Family history was significant for both mother and maternal grandmother with hypercholesterolemia on statin treatment. His grandmother had an early heart attack at age 40. On physical examination, his blood pressure and growth parameters were normal. The patient's BMI is at the 75th percentile for age. He did not have acanthosis or xanthomas.

Questions to consider:

- *Would you consider lipid screening for this patient?*
- *What laboratory abnormalities would indicate a need for medication therapy for him?*

Answer: The patient is between ages 9 and 11 years, and hence should undergo a non-fasting lipid screening based on the universal screening recommendations. He also has first/ second degree relative with premature cardiovascular disease which would have qualified him for selective lipid screening as well, had he been evaluated at a younger age. He does not appear to have any secondary conditions that predispose him for dyslipidemia

The lipid profile is shown below:
Total cholesterol: 280 mg/dL
Triglycerides: 90 mg/dL
LDL-C: 222 mg/dL

HDL-C: 40 mg/dL
Non-HDL-C: 240 mg/dL
Based on this lipid profile, he has heterozygous FH (LDL-C > 160 mg/dL and positive family history of premature CVD).

Question to consider: Would you consider screening other family members?

Answer: Based on recommendations for cascade screening, it is important to screen the siblings and father.

Conclusions

Universal pediatric lipid screening is currently recommended for all children and adolescents at ages 9–11, and again between the ages 17–21 years. Selective screening is recommended for children between the ages 2–8 and 12–16 years who have risk factors/risk conditions. Cascade screening is indicated if familial hypercholesterolemia is identified.

References

1. Hu P, et al. Prevalence of familial hypercholesterolemia among the general population and patients with atherosclerotic cardiovascular disease: a systematic review and meta-analysis. Circulation. 2020;141(22):1742–59.
2. Gooding HC, et al. Application of pediatric and adult guidelines for treatment of lipid levels among US adolescents transitioning to young adulthood. JAMA Pediatr. 2015;169(6):569–74.
3. de Ferranti SD, et al. Cardiovascular risk reduction in high-risk pediatric patients: a scientific statement from the American Heart Association. Circulation. 2019;139(13):e603–34.
4. Expert Panel on Integrated Guidelines for Cardiovascular Health and Risk Reduction in Children and Adolescents, National Heart, Lung, and Blood Institute. Expert panel on integrated guidelines for cardiovascular health and risk reduction in children and adolescents: summary report. Pediatrics. 2011;128(Suppl 5):S213–56.
5. Bradley CB, et al. Prevalence of high cholesterol, high blood pressure, and smoking among elementary schoolchildren in North Carolina. N C Med J. 1997;58(5):362–7.
6. Ned RM, Sijbrands EJ. Cascade screening for familial hypercholesterolemia (FH). PLoS Currents. 2011;3:RRN1238.
7. Cook S, Auinger P, Huang TT. Growth curves for cardio-metabolic risk factors in children and adolescents. J Pediatr. 2009;155(3):S6 e15–26.
8. American Academy of Pediatrics. National Cholesterol Education Program: report of the expert panel on blood cholesterol levels in children and adolescents. Pediatrics. 1992;89(3 Pt 2):525–84.
9. Stewart J, et al. Hyperlipidemia. Pediatr Rev. 2020;41(8):393–402.
10. Shah AS, Wilson DP. Primary hypertriglyceridemia in children and adolescents. J Clin Lipidol. 2015;9(5 Suppl):S20–8.

Chapter 4
Measurement of Lipids and Lipoproteins

Marissa Lightbourne and Stephanie T. Chung

Clinical Case
A 14-year-old girl presents to your afternoon diabetes clinic for routine follow-up of type 2 diabetes. The non-fasting lipid panel drawn the week before the visit shows total cholesterol of 240 mg/dL, triglycerides 644 mg/dL, HDL cholesterol 35 mg/dL, and LDL cholesterol was unable to be calculated. What is the next best step in the management?

A. Repeat lipid panel now and start statin therapy if total cholesterol is >200 mg/dL.
B. Start statin therapy now without additional laboratory tests.
C. Obtain lipoprotein (a) and direct LDL and if elevated start statin therapy.
D. Obtain a fasting lipid panel on two separate occasions at least 2 weeks apart.

Plasma Lipids

Accurate and precise assessments of plasma lipids are critical for the screening, diagnosis, and treatment/management of lipid disorders in pediatrics. Plasma lipids are classified by hydrated density or by migration on electrophoresis and include cholesterol (-C) and triglycerides (TG) that are transported in six [6] major lipoproteins: chylomicrons, very-low density lipoproteins (VLDL), intermediate-density

M. Lightbourne · S. T. Chung (✉)
Diabetes, Endocrinology, and Obesity Branch, National Institute of Diabetes & Digestive & Kidney Diseases, National Institutes of Health, Bethesda, MD, USA
e-mail: marissa.lightbourne@nih.gov; stephanie.chung@nih.gov

A. Ashraf, B. Sunil (eds.), *Pediatric Dyslipidemia*,
https://doi.org/10.1007/978-3-031-24113-0_4

lipoproteins (IDL), low-density lipoproteins (LDL), and high-density lipoproteins (HDL). Direct ultracentrifugation is the gold-standard technique for quantifying plasma lipids, but maybe expensive and time-consuming [1].

Standard Lipid Panel

Automated standardized enzymatic/spectrophotometric methods (standard lipid panel) are the main stay of plasma lipid assessment. These tests are obtained from a single serum sample and are convenient and cost-effective for routine clinical use with a coefficient of variation (CV) <5% [2, 3]. The standard lipid panel typically estimates five [5] plasma lipid concentrations; three [3] are directly measured (TG, total cholesterol [TC], and HDL-C) and two [2] are derived (LDL-C and non-HDL-C). Concentrations of VLDL-C may also be reported and are calculated based on the assumption that VLDL is composed of ~20% of TG [1]. In the United States, test performance and reliability of the standard lipid panel are assured by the Center for Disease Control and Prevention (CDC) Lipids Standardization Program (LSP) . The LSP monitors the accuracy of clinical and research laboratories by providing blinded LSP standards traceable to the CDC Reference laboratory for measuring TC, TG, and HDL-C. Of all the plasma lipids, LDL-C is the most ubiquitously used for diagnosing and monitoring lipid disorders in youth and adults [3, 4]. LDL-C is usually estimated from the standard lipid panel but can also be directly measured. A brief discussion of the assumptions and limitations of the two methods used to assess LDL-C is outlined below.

Estimated LDL-C

LDL-C is routinely estimated in clinical practice with the Friedewald equation (Table 4.1). This estimation is simple and accurate for quantifying the cholesterol contained in LDL particles and is based on three assumptions: (1) the ratio of TC:TG in VLDL-C is 4:1, (2) there are only modest elevations in TG concentrations, and (3) there is an equal distribution of VLDL in the serum sample. If these conditions are not met, for example, during the non-fasting state, when TG concentrations are ≥400 mg/dL, or LDL-C is <70 mg/dL, the equation underestimates LDL-C. Contemporary equations that account for greater TG variability (TG ≥400 mg/dL) and/ or when LDL-C is <70 mg/dL are now available for use (Table 4.1).

Table 4.1 Examples of commonly used equations for calculating LDL-C. All values are in mg/dL

Equation	Formula (LDL-C mg/dL)	Limitations
Friedewald [12]	$TC-(HDL-C)-\frac{TG}{5}$	Underestimates LDL-C when TG ≥400 mg/dL and LDL-C < 70 mg/dL
Martin-Hopkins [13]	$(nonHDL-C)-\left(\frac{TG}{Adjustable\ factor^{a}}\right)$	Overestimates LDL-C when TG ≥400 mg/dL and LDL-C >100 mg/dL
NIH [14]	$\frac{TC}{0.948}-\frac{HDL-C}{0.971}-\left(\frac{TG}{8.56}+\frac{TG\times \mathrm{Non-HDL-C}}{2140}-\frac{TG^{2}}{16100}\right)-9.44$	Needs validation in general pediatric population

LDL low-density lipoproteins, *TG* triglycerides, *HDL* high-density lipoproteins

[a] The adjustable factor is determined as the strata-specific median TG:VLDL-C ratio [13]

Table 4.2 Biological factors that may influence lipid concentrations

Factor	Description	Author/Year	Reference
Age	TC, LDL-C, and TG increase up to age 2 years, decline during adolescence and rise to adult levels by 18–19 years of age	Eissa et al. (2016)	[15, 16]
Puberty	During puberty TC, TG, and LDL-C decrease by ~10–20%.	Kwiterovich et al. (1997)	[17]
Biological sex	HDL-C concentrations decrease during puberty in males only	Jolliffe et al. (2006)	[16]
Race	African American compared to white children have higher levels of TC and HDL-C and lower levels of VLDL-C and TG	Sumner et al. (2009)	[18]
Diurnal variation	TG levels vary widely throughout the day and are lowest ~3–4 AM	Barter et al. (1971)	[19]

TC total cholesterol, *TG* triglycerides, *LDL-C* low-density lipoprotein—cholesterol, *HDL-C* high-density lipoprotein—cholesterol concentrations

Direct LDL-C Measurements

Direct LDL-C assays provide an alternative method for assessing LDL-C. The vertical-spin density gradient ultracentrifugation is the gold-standard method (CV: 1–2%), but other enzymatic/spectrophotometric methods, elimination-detergent, and direct homogenous assays are available. Most direct LDL-C assays are commercially available but are not routinely recommended because of lack of assay standardization and expense. Though the direct LDL-C has improved analytical performance compared to calculated LDL-C, the direct LDL-C assays also have reduced specificity in the presence of severe hypertriglyericidemia and markedly low HDL-C that limits its widespread use [5].

Special Considerations

Measuring LDL-C has revolutionized the field of cardiology and is widely used in clinical practice. Although the majority of atherogenic lipoproteins are LDL, measuring LDL-C does not estimate the total atherogenic risk associated with all apolipoprotein B (apoB) containing particles (chylomicrons, VLDL, and IDL). Total atherogenic risk is associated with the cholesterol content and the number of apoB particles that become trapped within the intima [6]. Other markers such as non-HDL-C or apoB concentrations give a global assessment of total atherogenic risk.

When interpreting the lipid panel, physiological and pathological factors should be considered. Table 4.2 outlines common physiologic variations in lipid parameters unique to the pediatric population. Obtaining a detailed medication history is also key because multiple medications may alter TG and LDL-C concentrations including, oral contraceptives, anti-hypertensives, steroids, antiviral therapies, anti-psychotics, retinoids, growth hormone, and immunosuppressants.

Expanded Lipid/Lipoprotein Profile

Expanded lipid/lipoprotein measurements provide detailed profiling of lipid parameters that are helpful in distinguishing between complex lipid disorders and may be useful for cardiovascular risk stratification. Two common methods are used for measuring the expanded lipid/lipoprotein profile: ultracentrifugation and nuclear magnetic resonance spectroscopy.

Vertical Spin Density Gradient Ultracentrifugation

The vertical autoprofile (VAP) test directly measures and routinely reports five lipoprotein classes and subclasses, including LDL-C, HDL-C, IDL, VLDL-C, and lipoprotein (a) and is unaffected by TG levels [7]. Further stratification of LDL pattern A, A/B, and B (representing large to small LDL) is possible with VAP ultracentrifugation and has been associated with increased cardiometabolic risk in youth. However, advanced lipoprotein testing with VAP is not widely available for clinical use, and VAP testing did not improve prediction for subclinical atherosclerosis in young adults [4].

Nuclear Magnetic Resonance Spectroscopy (NMR)

Nuclear magnetic resonance (NMR) spectroscopy measures the amplitudes of the lipid methyl group NMR signals to determine the lipoprotein particle size and number (-P). Lipoprotein subclasses (Fig. 4.1) are derived by deconvolution of the lipid methyl signal envelope contained within these spectra [8]. NMR lipoprotein particles are separated based on particle size only (Table 4.3). The TRL-P subclasses include triglyceride-rich containing lipids such as chylomicrons, chylomicron remnants, VLDL, and IDL. In the United States, analyses are typically conducted with a 400 Mhz proton NMR Profiler and Vantera Clinical Analyzer platforms using the lipid methyl signal envelope algorithm analysis and particle concentration reported in nmol/L.

This extended lipoprotein panel is not currently recommended in pediatrics though high concentrations of small LDL-P and total LDL-P were associated with increased cardiovascular risk in youth and are strong cardiovascular risk predictor in adults. There are no clinical studies evaluating the risk/benefit ratio of LDL-P

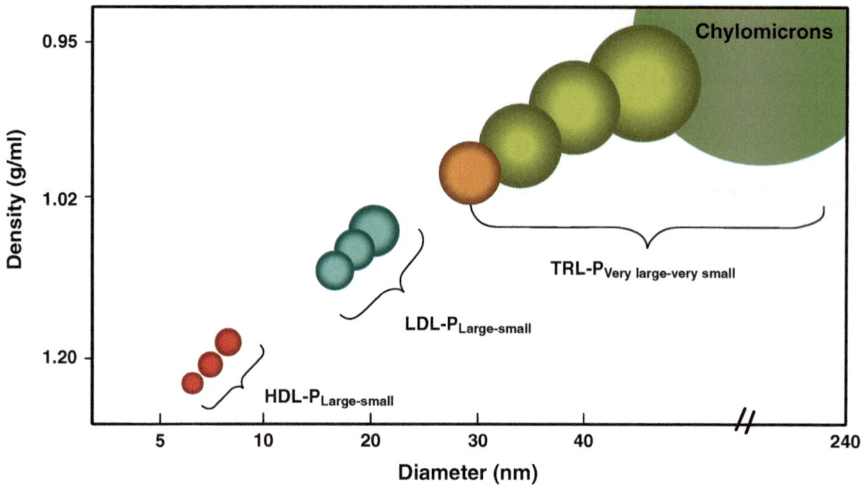

Fig. 4.1 Lipoprotein particle size and density. *LDL* low-density lipoproteins, *TG* triglycerides, *HDL* high-density lipoproteins

Table 4.3 Lipoprotein LP4 nuclear magnetic resonance MetaboProfile™ parameter diameter size estimates (not accounting for possible age variation in childhood)

Parameter	Diameter Estimate (nm)
Triglyceride-rich lipoprotein particle (TRL-P, nmol/L)	
Total TRL-P	24–240
Very large TRL-P	90–240
Large TRL-P	50–89
Medium TRL-P	37–49
Small TRL-P	30–36
Very small TRL-P	24–29
Low-density lipoprotein particles (LDL-P, nmol/L)	
Total LDL-P	19–23
Large LDL-P	21.5–23
Medium LDL-P	20.5–21.4
Small LDL-P	19–20.4
High-density lipoprotein particles (HDL-P, nmol/L)	
Total HDL-P	7.5–13
Large HDL-P	10.3–12.0
Medium HDL-P	8.7–9.5
Small HDL-P	7.4–7.8
Mean particle size (nm)	
TRL-P	30–100
LDL-P	19–22.5
HDL-P	7.4–13

TRL-P triglyceride-rich lipoprotein particle, *LDL-P* low-density lipoprotein particles, *HDL-P* high-density lipoprotein particles assessment in youth for predicting cardiovascular disease later in life. Large studies are needed to determine normative data for lipoprotein concentrations in diverse populations and across the pubertal spectrum and its utility as a screening and diagnostic tool for hyperlipidemic disorders is under investigation.

Apolipoprotein B (apoB)

Apolipoprotein B is the principal apolipoprotein in chylomicrons, chylomicron remnants, VLDL, LDL, and lipoprotein (a). Each of these particles contain one apoB molecule: apolipoprotein B-48 (apoB-48) in chylomicrons and its remnants and apolipoprotein B-100 in VLDL, LDL, and lipoprotein (a). Immunoassays are commercially available to measure total apoB, and these tests can be done in the fasting or non-fasting state. Direct immunoassay measurements of apoB-100 and intestinally derived apob-48 are used in research, but their clinical applicability is uncertain.

In adults, elevated apoB concentrations reflect the cumulative risk of all apoB containing particles (VLDL, LDL, and IDL) and are strong indicators of cardiovascular disease compared to LDL-C. Discordantly high apoB concentrations with low-normal LDL-C and non-HDL-C is a marker of cardiovascular disease in adults. Normative values and cut-points for apoB in children were empirically derived from the Third National Health and Nutrition Examination Survey (1988–1994) (NHANES III), but there was no clear advantage of using apoB over LDL-C when screening for dyslipidemia [4]. Disadvantages of measuring apoB in pediatrics include the high assay cost, analytical variability, and non-superiority for risk-prediction compared to non-HDL cholesterol.

Lipoprotein (a)

Lipoprotein (a) [Lp(a)] is a cholesterol-rich lipoprotein—similar in composition to LDL, consisting of a unique apolipoprotein, apo(a). Lipoprotein (a) has homology to plasminogen and inhibits fibrinolysis. It can be detected by electrophoresis and immunoblot staining as a band midway between pre-beta and beta bands [9]. A variety of immunoassays are commercially available to quantify Lp(a), but there is a lack of standardized assays that limits its clinical utility. Preferred immunoassays are monoclonal and account for variability in isoform size, if not the assay may over or underestimate concentration [10]. Enzymatic assays that are isoform insensitive and measure lipoprotein(a) in nmol/L are more specific, but their widespread use in clinical practice has not been uniformly adopted, especially in pediatrics. In children, high Lp(a) concentrations were associated with impaired endothelial function, but the clinical utility for predicting future cardiovascular risk is yet uncertain. Lp(a) may increase on statin therapy.

Other Lipid-Related Assays

Apolipoprotein A1

Apolipoprotein A-I (ApoA-I), the major apolipoprotein component of HDL is a multifunctional protein, involved in cholesterol traffic and inflammation. The immunoassay may be collected at any time of day (non-fasting). Normative values and cut-points for children were empirically derived from the Third National Health and Nutrition Examination Survey (1988–1994) (NHANES III). In youth, apoA-I was associated with cardiovascular risk, but there are no clinical guidelines for its use. In general, apoA-I is prone to catabolism especially in hypertriglyceridemic states, making HDL-C the preferred measure of HDL.

NMR-Derived Marker Lipoprotein Insulin Resistance Index (LP-IR)

The LP-IR index is a marker derived from the NMR lipoprotein profile that was designed to estimate insulin sensitivity and diabetes risk. The index is a composite score of six lipoprotein parameters: large VLDL-P number, VLDL size, small LDL-P number, LDL size, large HDL-P number, and HDL size [11]. The score ranges from 0 (insulin sensitive) to 100 (insulin resistant) and was developed and validated based on fasting and insulin clamp-derived measures of insulin resistance [11]. The LP-IR index is measured on an automated nuclear magnetic resonance (NMR) clinical analyzer using LabCorp's proprietary Vantera® platform [11].

The LP-IR can be obtained from the same fasting sample used to assess the lipid and extended lipoprotein profile. Despite extensive research on the use of NMR profiles in pediatric populations, data in LP-IR are sparse in youth, and it is not clinically recommended. Observational cross-sectional studies indicate LP-IR maybe a robust indicator of insulin resistance in healthy children as well as those with obesity and abnormal glucose tolerance. The theoretical advantage to using an automated score is the enhanced simplicity and convenience of assessing insulin resistance and risk for diabetes prior to the development of hyperglycemia. Large prospective studies are needed to confirm the LP-IR index clinical utility and widespread applicability for predicting type 2 diabetes in youth and older adults.

Clinical Case
Answer D

According to AAP/NCEP 2011 recommendations, a non-fasting lipid profile is a valid screening test for hyperlipidemia [4]. When lipid parameters are elevated, the next step for the diagnosis and management is to obtain two [2] fasting lipid panels at least 2 weeks apart and average the lipid parameters. Guidelines for diet/lifestyle and pharmacotherapy are primarily based on risk stratification using a detailed family and personal history and fasting LDL-C concentrations [4].

Clinical Case Follow-Up

The repeat fasting lipid panel showed total cholesterol 198 mg/dL, triglycerides 420 mg/dL, and HDL cholesterol 33 mg/dL, LDL cholesterol could not be calculated. What is the next step in evaluation?

A. Calculate non-HDL cholesterol and repeat the fasting lipid panel.
B. Start statin therapy now.
C. Obtain lipoprotein (a) and direct LDL and if elevated start statin therapy.
D. Obtain extended lipoprotein panel and start statin therapy if LDL particle number is >1000 nmol/L.

Answer A

As per clinical guidelines, a second fasting lipid panel is needed for diagnosis and to guide management [4]. When LDL-C cannot be calculated, non-HDL-C and TG should be assessed. Individuals with a non-HDL cholesterol of ≥145 mg/dL should be referred to a lipid specialist for consideration of lipid-lowering therapy (e.g., statin) [4]. Alternative equations can also be used to estimate LDL-C and direct LDL assays may be useful but are not recommended due to their high cost and lack of assay standardization. Normative values for apoB in children are available but current guidelines do not utilize apoB thresholds for guiding management [4]. Measurements of lipoprotein (a) and an extended lipoprotein panel are research tools that are not recommended in the routine management of metabolic dyslipidemia in youth except in youth who have a personal history of stroke or have a strong family history of early cardiovascular death [4].

Acknowledgments None.

Funding STC and ML are supported by the Intramural Program of National Institute of Diabetes & Digestive & Kidney Diseases at the National Institutes of Health in Bethesda, MD.

References

1. Friedewald WT, Levy RI, Fredrickson DS. Estimation of the concentration of low-density lipoprotein cholesterol in plasma, without use of the preparative ultracentrifuge. Clin Chem. 1972;18(6):499–502.
2. McNamara JR, Schaefer EJ. Automated enzymatic standardized lipid analyses for plasma and lipoprotein fractions. Clin Chim Acta. 1987;166(1):1–8.
3. Grundy SM, Stone NJ, Bailey AL, Beam C, Birtcher KK, Blumenthal RS, et al. 2018 AHA/ACC/AACVPR/AAPA/ABC/ACPM/ADA/AGS/APhA/ASPC/NLA/PCNA guideline on the management of blood cholesterol: a report of the American College of Cardiology/American Heart Association Task Force on Clinical Practice Guidelines. J Am Coll Cardiol. 2018;139:e1082–143.
4. Expert Panel on Integrated Guidelines for Cardiovascular Health and Risk Reduction in Children and Adolescents, National Heart, Lung, and Blood Institute. Expert panel on integrated guidelines for cardiovascular health and risk reduction in children and adolescents: summary report. Pediatrics. 2011;128 Suppl 5(Suppl 5):S213–56.
5. Miller WG, Myers GL, Sakurabayashi I, Bachmann LM, Caudill SP, Dziekonski A, et al. Seven direct methods for measuring HDL and LDL cholesterol compared with ultracentrifugation reference measurement procedures. Clin Chem. 2010;56(6):977–86.
6. Sniderman AD, Thanassoulis G, Glavinovic T, Navar AM, Pencina M, Catapano A, et al. Apolipoprotein B particles and cardiovascular disease: a narrative review. JAMA Cardiol. 2019;4:1287.
7. Kulkarni KR. Cholesterol profile measurement by vertical auto profile method. Clin Lab Med. 2006;26(4):787–802.
8. Matyus SP, Braun PJ, Wolak-Dinsmore J, Jeyarajah EJ, Shalaurova I, Xu Y, et al. NMR measurement of LDL particle number using the Vantera clinical analyzer. Clin Biochem. 2014;47(16–17):203–10.
9. Kawakami K, Tsukada A, Okubo M, Tsukada T, Kobayashi T, Yamada N, et al. A rapid electrophoretic method for the detection of serum Lp(a) lipoprotein. Clin Chim Acta. 1989;185(2):147–55.
10. Marcovina SM, Albers JJ, Scanu AM, Kennedy H, Giaculli F, Berg K, et al. Use of a reference material proposed by the International Federation of Clinical Chemistry and Laboratory Medicine to evaluate analytical methods for the determination of plasma lipoprotein(a). Clin Chem. 2000;46(12):1956–67.
11. Shalaurova I, Connelly MA, Garvey WT, Otvos JD. Lipoprotein insulin resistance index: a lipoprotein particle-derived measure of insulin resistance. Metab Syndr Relat Disord. 2014;12(8):422–9.
12. Tremblay AJ, Morrissette H, Gagne JM, Bergeron J, Gagne C, Couture P. Validation of the Friedewald formula for the determination of low-density lipoprotein cholesterol compared with beta-quantification in a large population. Clin Biochem. 2004;37(9):785–90.
13. Martin SS, Blaha MJ, Elshazly MB, Toth PP, Kwiterovich PO, Blumenthal RS, et al. Comparison of a novel method vs the Friedewald equation for estimating low-density lipoprotein cholesterol levels from the standard lipid profile. JAMA. 2013;310(19):2061–8.
14. Sampson M, Ling C, Sun Q, Harb R, Ashmaig M, Warnick R, et al. A new equation for calculation of low-density lipoprotein cholesterol in patients with normolipidemia and/or hypertriglyceridemia. JAMA Cardiol. 2020;5:540.
15. Eissa MA, Mihalopoulos NL, Holubkov R, Dai S, Labarthe DR. Changes in fasting lipids during puberty. J Pediatr. 2016;170:199–205.
16. Jolliffe CJ, Janssen I. Distribution of lipoproteins by age and gender in adolescents. Circulation. 2006;114(10):1056–62.

17. Kwiterovich PO Jr, Barton BA, McMahon RP, Obarzanek E, Hunsberger S, Simons-Morton D, et al. Effects of diet and sexual maturation on low-density lipoprotein cholesterol during puberty: the dietary intervention study in children (DISC). Circulation. 1997;96(8):2526–33.
18. Sumner AE. Ethnic differences in triglyceride levels and high-density lipoprotein lead to underdiagnosis of the metabolic syndrome in black children and adults. J Pediatr. 2009;155(3):S7 e7–11.
19. Barter PJ, Carroll KF, Nestel PJ. Diurnal fluctuations in triglyceride, free fatty acids, and insulin during sucrose consumption and insulin infusion in man. J Clin Invest. 1971;50(3):583–91.

Chapter 5
Diagnosis and Management of Youth with Disorders of LDL Cholesterol

Adam L. Ware and Don P. Wilson

Introduction

The majority of cholesterol in the circulation is transported within low-density lipoproteins (LDL), and data from epidemiologic, genetic, and interventional studies has clearly demonstrated its causal role in atherosclerotic cardiovascular disease (ASCVD). As a result, the estimated or directly measured cholesterol content of LDL (i.e. LDL-C) plays a prominent role in screening and therapeutic recommendations of both adults and children. The pathophysiology of ASCVD, however, is complex and influenced by a variety of additional causative and enhancing factors in addition to the quantity of LDL-C within the circulation (Fig. 5.1). Nonetheless, abnormalities in lipoprotein metabolism which increase LDL-C represent approximately 50% of the population attributable risk of ASCVD.

In addition to its cholesterol content, the nature of the LDL particle, including its size, density, and number contributes to the development of ASCVD. LDL particles typically vary in size (18–25 nm) and density (1.019–1.063 g/mL); small dense LDL particles (sdLDL) being more atherogenic than those that are larger and less dense.

The composition and quantity of LDL particles and their cholesterol content is influenced by multiple factors, including heredity, environment, and other medical conditions. Alterations in LDL-C content in combination with other biomarkers, clinical history, and genetic testing can help determine the underlying etiology. In

A. L. Ware
Department of Pediatric Cardiology, University of Utah, Salt Lake City, UT, USA
e-mail: adam.ware@hsc.utah.edu

D. P. Wilson (✉)
Department of Pediatric Endocrinology and Diabetes, Cook Children's Medical Center, Fort Worth, TX, USA
e-mail: don.wilson@cookchildrens.org

A. Ashraf, B. Sunil (eds.), *Pediatric Dyslipidemia*,
https://doi.org/10.1007/978-3-031-24113-0_5

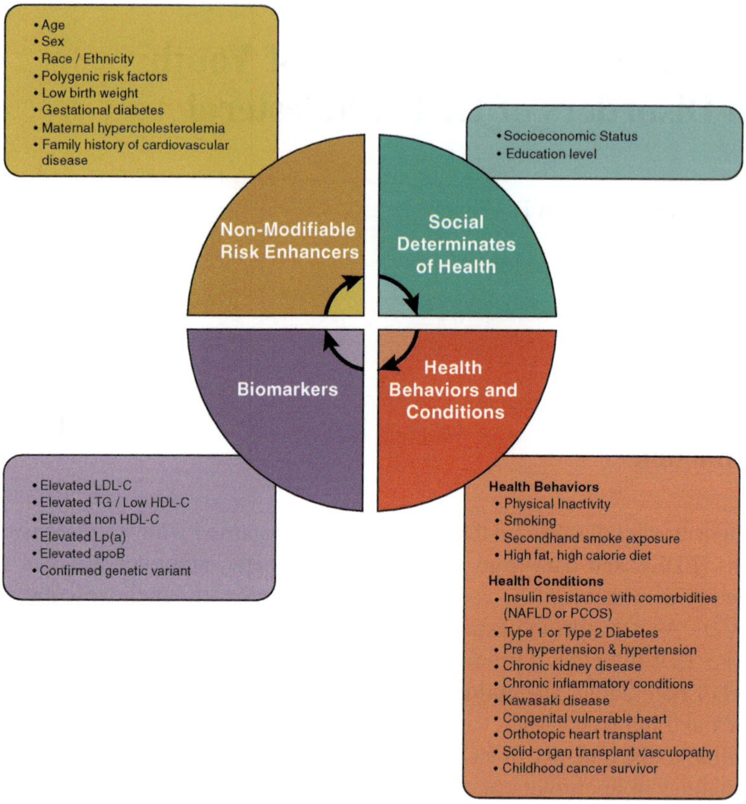

Fig. 5.1 Global risk factors for atherosclerotic cardiovascular disease. Source: Amy L. Peterson, Catherine J. McNeal, and Don P. Wilson. Prevention of Atherosclerotic Cardiovascular Disease in Children with Familial Hypercholesterolemia. Current Atherosclerosis Reports

this chapter, we provide an overview of LDL specific abnormalities in cholesterol metabolism, discuss interpretation of lipid test results, and provide recommendations for timely interventions, which are safe and effective in children.

Hypercholesterolemia

Overview

Hypercholesterolemia is common in children, although the vast majority are asymptomatic. Current U.S. guidelines recommend targeted cholesterol screening of children 2 years-of-age and older, and universal screening beginning at 9–11 years-of-age [1].

A fasting or non-fasting lipid panel can be utilized for screening, but guidelines suggest that cholesterol levels be averaged from two separate fasting lipid panels to confirm an abnormal result. Screening may identify isolated elevations of cholesterol in specific lipoprotein classes or combinations of abnormalities. The pattern of dyslipidemia is often helpful in determining the mostly likely cause.

Lipid and lipoprotein levels in children are generally defined using age specific mean values in the general population. The National Health and Nutrition Examination Surveys (NHANES) reported a mean LDL-C level of 88 mg/dL in adolescents 12–19 years, with Asians and Blacks having the highest levels. Overall, elevated levels of LDL-C were present in 5.5% of males and 7.5% of females in the population [2]. Acceptable and elevated levels of lipids for youth are shown in Table 5.1.

Causes of elevated LDL-C may be acquired (Table 5.2), genetic (Table 5.3) or both. A detailed physical examination, clinical history, and family history are essential in the initial diagnosis. A careful evaluation for secondary causes of elevated LDL-C is the first step in evaluating an abnormal lipid profile. Several common pediatric medications such as isotretinoin, atypical antipsychotics, and oral contraceptives are well known to cause dyslipidemia, including elevations of LDL-C. Obesity is a major risk factor for dyslipidemia, and approximately 60–70% of obese children have an abnormal lipid panel [3]. Combined dyslipidemia of obesity (CDO) is commonly identified as a result of lipid screening. CDO is characterized by elevated triglycerides (TG) and low high-density lipoprotein cholesterol (HDL-C). Non-HDL-C is generally elevated with normal to mildly elevated LDL-C. While the absolute elevation in LDL-C may be low, the LDL particles are smaller, denser, and more numerous. The increased risk of ASCVD in CDO is associated with high levels of sdLDL particles, increased oxidation of lipids, and enhanced permeability of the arterial wall.

Table 5.1 Acceptable, borderline, and high plasma lipid, lipoprotein, and apolipoprotein concentrations for children and adolescents. Adapted from Expert Panel on Integrated Guidelines for Cardiovascular Health and Risk Reduction in Children and Adolescents, National Heart, Lung, and Blood Institute. Expert panel on integrated guidelines for cardiovascular health and risk reduction in children and adolescents: Summary report. *Pediatrics*. 2011; 128 (Suppl 5): S213–S256

Category	Acceptable	Borderline	High	Low
Total cholesterol	<170 mg/dL	170–199 mg/dL	≥200 mg/dL	–
LDL cholesterol	<110 mg/dL	110–129 mg/dL	≥130 mg/dL	–
Non-HDL cholesterol	<120 mg/dL	120–144 mg/dL	≥145 mg/dL	–
Triglycerides				
0–9 years	<75 mg/dL	75–99 mg/dL	≥100 mg/dL	–
10–19 years	<90 mg/dL	90–129 mg/dL	≥130 mg/dL	–
HDL cholesterol	>45 mg/dL	40–45 mg/dL	–	<40 mg/dL

HDL high-density lipoprotein, *LDL* low-density lipoprotein

To convert milligrams per deciliter to millimoles per liter for cholesterol levels, multiply 0.0259. To convert milligrams per deciliter to millimoles per liter for triglyceride levels, multiply by 0.0113

Low cutoff points for HDL cholesterol represents approximately the tenth percentile. The cutoff points for high and borderline-high values represent approximately the 95th and 75th percentiles, respectively

Table 5.2 Secondary causes of elevated LDL cholesterol

Medications	Endocrine	Renal	Hepatic	Infectious	Genetic	Environmental
Corticosteroids Isotretinoin Oral contraceptives Antiretrovirals Atypical antipsychotics	Hypothyroidism Diabetes Cushing's syndrome Growth hormone deficiency	Nephrotic syndrome Chronic renal disease	Alagille syndrome Cholestasis Hepatitis Hemolytic uremic syndrome	Acute infection	Gaucher disease Glycogen storage Disease	Alcohol Anorexia Obesity Pregnancy

Table 5.3 Genetic causes of LDL-C abnormalities

Condition	Frequency	Involved genes	Common lipid abnormalities			Xanthoma	ASCVD risk
			LDL-C	HDL-C	TG		
FCH	1–2% of population	Polygenic	↑ or ↑↑	↓	↑↑	No	↑ or ↑↑
FH	Polygenic 1:20	Polygenic	↑ or ↑↑	-	-	No	↑ or ↑↑
	Heterozygous 1:200	*LDLR* *APOB* *PCKS9*	↑↑	-	-	Adult	↑↑
	Homozygous 1:1M		↑↑↑	-	-	Child	↑↑↑
Sitosterolemia	1:50,000	*ABCG5* *ABCG8*	Nl to ↑↑↑	-	-	Adult	↑↑
LAL-D	1:40,000–1:300,000	*LIPA*	↑ to ↑↑	↓	↑	No	↑
CTX	1:36,000–1:468,000	*CYP27A1*	Nl to ↓	↓	↑	Child	↑↑

The most common inherited forms of dyslipidemia occur due to the interaction of several contributing gene variants along with environmental triggers

FCH familial combined hyperlipidemia, *FH* familial hypercholesterolemia, *LAL-D* lysosomal acid lipase deficiency, *CTX* cerebrotendinous xanthomatosis

LDL-C = low-density lipoprotein cholesterol, HDL-C = high-density lipoprotein cholesterol, TG = triglyceride, ASCVD = atheroscerolic cardiovascular disease

Once acquired causes have been eliminated or optimally managed, genetic variants should be considered. The classic genetic etiology for elevated LDL-C is familial hypercholesterolemia (FH). Heterozygous hypercholesterolemia (HeFH), an autosomal co-dominant genetic disorder, is very common (1 in 200–300); while the more severe homozygous disease (HoFH) is rare (1 in 300,000–1,000,000). Both are characterized by impaired cholesterol metabolism of varying severity. The most common variant for FH is in the gene for the LDL receptor. Less commonly, variants are present in genes encoding the LDL receptor ligand (apolipoprotein B), LDL receptor regulating enzyme (PCSK9), or LDL receptor adaptor protein-1 (LDLRAP1). FH typically presents as an isolated elevation in LDL-C, often with a family history of premature ASCVD-related events, such as angina, myocardial infarction, and stroke (Table 5.3). Early ASCVD is defined as occurring in men <55 years-of-age; women <65. The degree to which LDL-C is elevated is a function of the unique gene variant, with levels ranging from 100–400 mg/dL in heterozygous and 400–1000 mg/dL in homozygous individuals with FH. Mutations that result in monogenic disease exhibit significant variability in phenotype and associated risk, including amongst carriers within the same family and carriers of the same mutation within different populations [4]. FH and other independent causes of dyslipidemia may co-exist. For example, individuals may have both CDO and FH, with lipid panels that demonstrate elevated TGs, low HDL-C, and elevated LDL-C.

Other genetic variants (Table 5.3) may mimic FH, and further testing may be necessary to identify these conditions. Sitosterolemia (phytosterolemia), an abnormality of adenosine triphosphate binding cassette transporter genes (*ABCG5, ABCG8*), leads to hyperabsorption of plant sterols and cholesterol in the intestines. It is associated with elevated ASCVD risk but, unlike FH, is characterized by elevated plasma sterol levels. Lysosomal acid lipase deficiency (Wolman's/cholesterol ester storage disease), an abnormality of the *LIPA* gene, causes accumulation of TGs and cholesterol esters in hepatic lysosomes. Affected children present with elevated LDL-C similar to those with FH, along with hepatomegaly, abnormal liver enzymes and high levels of TGs accompanied by low HDL-C.

Diagnosis

Biochemical Testing

A standard lipid profile (TC, TG, HDL-C and LDL-C) plays an important role in evaluating cardiovascular disease risk. LDL-C is generally a calculated value, which is invalid when TG exceed 400 mg/dL. In cases of elevated TG, LDL-C should be measured directly. Tables 5.2 and 5.3 list many of the most common causes of elevated LDL-C. Secondary causes such as medications and disorders of the thyroid (free T4 and TSH), liver (AST/ALT), and kidney (BUN/Cr and UA) should be excluded prior to considering genetic variants, although some children may have multiple causes.

Advanced lipid testing, which measures LDL particle number, size, and density, is not routinely recommended; although it may be helpful when clinical history, particularly family history, and laboratory test results are discordant. In children who are obese, the TG/HDL-C ratio provides additional insight. An elevated TG/HDL level ($\geq$3 in whites; $\geq$2.5 in blacks) is associated with increased levels of atherogenic TG-rich lipoprotein remnants, including sdLDL [5]. Since all atherogenic lipoproteins, including lipoprotein(a) [Lp(a)] contain a single apolipoprotein B (apoB), this measurement provides an excellent estimate of ASCVD risk. Measurement of apoB is particularly helpful in children who are receiving lipid-lowering medications, since levels may be discordant when compared to LDL-C. Derived from a standard lipid profile, a calculated non-HDL-C (TC—HDL-C) provides an estimate of apoB, without additional blood sampling or cost as further explained in Chap. 4.

Genetic Testing

Genetic testing in individuals with clinically suspected FH provides valuable insight into phenotype-genotype correlations. Population studies have shown that variants that result in monogenic disease exhibit significant variability in phenotype and associated risk, either in carriers within the same family or among carriers of the same variant within different populations. Over 100 genes have been identified that may have a direct impact on lipid levels, resulting in complex interactions between genes and resultant phenotypes. Variants of unknown significance (VUS) add complexity to the interpretation of genetic results and require phenotypic correlation. While genetic testing may provide useful information for risk stratification, genetic counselling is needed to help children and parents understand the implication of the diagnosis and aid in clinical decision-making. An overview of genetic testing in clinical practice is shown in Table 5.4. The implications of a genetic diagnosis, including VUS, treatment options, potential for psychological harm, stigmatization, and discrimination should also be discussed (Table 5.5) [6].

Table 5.4 Genetic testing for FH—clinical considerations

Prior to testing:

- Screen for secondary causes of hypercholestolemia (thyroid, liver, kidney) and medications that increase LDL-C
- Obtain a detailed family history of early ASCVD focusing on: Men <55 and women <65 years old with hypercholesterolemia use of lipid-lowering medications, a history of CVD events (angina, myocardial infarction, stoke), or CVD interventions (percutaneous coronary intervention, coronary artery bypass grafting)
- Provide detailed counseling including a discussion of benefits and potential harms (Table 5.4):
  - Type of genetic test(s) to be performed
  - Implications with regard to recommendations for use of lipid-lowering medications
  - Potential denial of coverage for genetic testing by the patient's insurance company
  - Potential impact of genetic testing in regard to insurance premiums or eligibility for life or long-term care insurance
  - Potential test results and implications of each in clinical decision-making and genetic counseling (see below)

Testing

- Test for suspected FH should include analysis of LDLR, APOB and PCSK9
- One time testing of Lp(a) is recommended in children with clinically suspected or genetically confirmed FH
- Routine measurement of apo B, apo A1, and advanced lipoprotein analysis is not routinely recommended (one or more may be helpful in selected cases)
- Screening of all non-modifiable and modifiable risk factors and risk enhancers. (Fig. 5.1)

After testing

- Provide post-test counseling, based upon the genetic test results, which includes

Positive	**Indeterminate**	**Negative**
Known or likely pathogenic variant	Variant of uncertain significance	No pathogenic variant identified

Table 5.4 (continued)

• Describes the specific type of pathogenic variant and its severity/risk of future ASCVD • Null variants are more adverse than defective variants • LDLR variants are more adverse than APOB and PCSK9 variants	• A variation in a genetic sequence for which the association with disease risk is unclear • A VUS should not be used in clinical decision-making • If a patient is identified to have a VUS, all clinical decisions should be based on personal and family history and not on the presence of the VUS • As more evidence becomes available, variants can be re-classified	• Consider alternative molecular etiologies and phenocopies: – Autosomal recessive FH (biallelic LDLRAP1 – Polygenic (up to 30% with FH) – High Lp(a) – *APOE* – Sitosterolemia (autosomal recessive pathogenic variants in ABCG5 or ABCG8) – Lysosomal acid lipase deficiency (autosomal recessive pathogenic variants in *LIPA*)
Cascade screening:		
Recommended. • Patients should be encouraged to share results with at-risk family members • Use of LDL-C levels to screen first degree relatives is not reliable because of the overlap between LDL-C levels in those with and without HeFH	Consider based on phenotype, family history, and identified VUS	Cascade screening: Based on results of additional diagnostic testing

Table 5.5 Potential benefits and harms of predictive genetic testing of children. Adapted from: Ethical and Policy Issues in Genetic Testing and Screening of Children. Pediatrics 2013; 131:620–622

Medical	
Benefits	Possibility of evolving therapeutic interventions, targeted surveillance, refinement of prognosis, and clarification of diagnosis
Harms	Misdiagnosis to the extent that genotype does not correlate with phenotype, ambiguous results in which a specific phenotype cannot be predicted and use of ineffective or harmful preventive or therapeutic interventions
Psychosocial	
Benefits	Reduction of uncertainty and anxiety, the opportunity for psychological adjustment, the ability to make realistic life plans, and sharing the information with family members
Harms	Alteration of self-image, distortion of parental perception of the child, increased anxiety and guilt, altered expectation by self and others, familial stress related to identification of other at-risk family members, difficulty obtaining life and/or disability insurance, and the detection of misattributed parentage
Reproductive	
Benefits	Avoiding the birth of a child with genetic disease or having time to prepare for the birth of a child with genetic disease
Harms	Changing family-planning decisions on the basis of social pressures

Imaging

The need for cardiovascular testing is based on the diagnosis. Cardiovascular imaging at diagnosis is primarily indicated in children with HoFH and includes an electrocardiogram, echocardiogram, age-appropriate stress testing, and advanced coronary artery imaging.

Non-invasive testing may play a role in other conditions associated with elevated LDL-C as well and can help assess the presence of subclinical atherosclerosis. Historically many of these non-invasive modalities have been utilized primary in research. Outcome studies in children are largely dependent on changes in markers of subclinical disease due to the manifestation of ASCVD-related outcomes, such as death or myocardial infarction, being age related. Assessment of subclinical atherosclerosis has allowed researchers to identify the impact of various risk factors and to track results of interventional studies. These techniques include:

Carotid Intima-Media Thickness (CIMT)

Assesses the thickness of the vascular intima and media layers within the carotid arteries. Intimal and medial thickening due to subclinical atherosclerosis can be measured and progression or regression of atherosclerosis over time can be evaluated. Patients with elevated LDL-C, such as those with FH, have been shown to have increased thickness of these layers. Additionally, CIMT thickness has been shown to regress following lipid-lowering treatment initiated at a young age.

Pulse Wave Velocity (PWV)

Tests arterial stiffness by measuring the velocity of blood in the descending aorta using a pressure sensor at the carotid and femoral artery. Increased stiffness in the aorta is caused by traditional ASCVD risk factors including elevated LDL-C. Higher PWV is an independent predictor of myocardial infarction in the Framingham study and can be accurately and reliably measured in children. Pulse wave analysis can also assess characteristics of the waveform itself.

Flow Mediated Dilation (FMD)

Measures the vascular response to ischemia (reactive hyperemia). This test assesses endothelial function and nitric oxide mediated vasodilation. A cuff is inflated in an upper extremity to a pressure exceeding the systolic BP. Blood vessel diameter and blood flow velocity are measured before and after occlusion and the percent change from baseline reported. A reduced change from baseline is consistent with endothelial dysfunction.

Echocardiograph

An "Echo" has become a standard tool for assessment of cardiac function. Subclinical valvular disease has been associated with severe elevations in LDL-C and progressive insufficiency of the aortic and mitral valves documented using this technique. Characteristics of the ascending aorta can also be evaluated including progressive supravalvar stenosis and plaque burden. In addition, echocardiography has been used to evaluate the epicardial adipose tissue, demonstrating an association between traditional CVD risk factors and epicardial fat thickness.

Advanced Imaging

Computerized Tomographic (CT) scans can be used to assess narrowing in the coronary artery lumen. This technique can also measure coronary artery calcium, although less utilized in children due to the lack of calcium deposition, which generally occurs later in life, and radiation exposure. Magnetic resonance imaging (MRI) scans can help define coronary artery anatomy, identify arterial narrowing, and assess myocardial perfusion. This technique is generally reserved for children with known or suspected coronary artery aneurysms, such as those with Kawasaki disease or congenital coronary artery abnormalities, and for follow-up after surgical manipulation or reimplantation of the coronary arteries.

Management

Interventions for children with elevated LDL-C, which are safe and effective, include therapeutic lifestyle changes (TLC) as well as lipid-lowering medications, most commonly statins**.** TLC is an essential component of treatment regardless of the underlying etiology and should be emphasized at each visit. A detailed history of the child's nutritional intake and usual level of activity should be documented. Guidance should be tailored to the needs of the family and the underlying cause of LDL-C elevation. When available, the assistance of a trained registered dietitian nutritionist is helpful. If TLC alone does not achieve the desired LDL-C level, pharmacologic interventions should be considered. TLC and lipid-lowering medication may sometimes be initiated concurrently [7]. Statins are the most used medications for children with persistently elevated levels of LDL-C. The safety and effectiveness of statin therapy has been demonstrated in multiple pediatric studies. All commercially available statins are FDA approved with pravastatin, rosuvastatin, and pitavastatin starting at age 8 and all others at age 10 for treatment of persistently elevated LDL-C ≥160 mg/dL after 3–6 months of lifestyle modification and a clinical picture consistent with FH [8]. While statins are generally very well tolerated in children, the side effect profile is similar to adults and families should be counseled on the possibility of myositis/myopathy and increases in transaminase levels. Reproductive age females should be cautioned regarding possible teratogenic effects, and contraception offered, if appropriate.

Table 5.6 Treatment for homozygous and heterozygous familial hypercholesterolemia

Homozygous Familial Hypercholesterolemia (HoFH)	Heterozygous Familial Hypercholesterolemia (HeFH)
Diagnosis **Clinical:** Untreated LDL-C ≥400 mg/dL Plus 1 additional criterion: • Biochemical or genetic evidence of FH in the biologic parents • Tendon xanthoma before age 10 • Aortic valve disease before age 20 **Genetic:** Confirmation of biallelic pathologic gene variants *(LDLR, APOB, PCSK9, LDLRAP1)* • Homozygous FH: Identical gene variants • Compound heterozygous FH: Non-identical gene variants	**Diagnosis** **Clinical:** LDL-C ≥160 mg/dL (children); ≥190 mg/dL (adults) Plus 1 additional criterion: • LDL-C suggestive of FH in a first degree relative • Family history of premature CAD • Family history of known pathogenic gene variant **Genetic:** • Confirmation of monoallelic variant *(LDLR, APOB, PCSK9, LDLRAP1)*
Treatment LDL-C goal: ≤100 mg/dL; ≤70 mg/dL with clinical CVD **At diagnosis:** • Therapeutic lifestyle changes • High intensity statin • LDL apheresis every 1–2 weeks **Adjunct therapies:** • Ezetimibe • Bile acid sequestrant • PCSK9 inhibitor • ANGPTL3 inhibitor **Other therapies:** • Niacin • Bempedoic acid • Lomitapide **Surgical therapies:** • Liver transplant	**Treatment** LDL-C goal: ≤130 mg/dL; or ≤100 mg/dL with additional risk factors **At diagnosis:** • Therapeutic lifestyle changes • Statin titrated to achieve goal **Adjunct therapies:** • Ezetimibe • Bile acid sequestrant • PCKS9 inhibitor **Other therapies:** • Niacin • Bempedoic acid • Lomitapide

Therapeutic lifestyle changes which include a low-fat, appropriate carbohydrate diet, weight loss if overweight or obese, participation in 30–60 min of moderate-to-vigorous physical activity per day and smoking avoidance or cessation should be encouraged in all children, including those who are prescribed lipid-lowering medication

All commercially available statins are FDA approved with pravastatin, rosuvastatin, and pitavastatin starting at age 8 and all others at age 10

Cascade screening should be recommended to all first-degree relatives (parents, siblings, and children) of an FH index case, followed by testing of second- and third-degree relatives if any of the first-degree relatives are affected. The most practical approach to cascade screening is biochemical testing of cholesterol, which is inexpensive and readily available. However, up to 25% of family members may be misdiagnosed as being either affected or unaffected when screening is based on cholesterol levels alone. Testing for a known genetic variant in the family combined with LDL-C levels will yield a definitive diagnosis

LDL-C low-density lipoprotein cholesterol, *CAH* coronary artery disease, *LDLR* low-density lipoprotein receptor, *APOB* apolipoprotein B, *PCSK9* proprotein convertase subtilisin/kexin type 9, *LDLRAP1* low-density lipoprotien receptor adaptor protein-1, *ANGPTL3* Angiopoietin-like 3 protein

Table 5.7 Novel therapeutic agents for lowering low-density lipoprotein cholesterol

Therapeutic targets for LDL-C lowering		
Site of action	Medications	Mechanism of action
Intestine	Ezetimibe Colesevelem	Blocks the internalization of the NPC1L1/ cholesterol complex Binds bile acids, prevents reabsorption and reduces cholesterol stores
Liver	Statins Bempedoic acid	HMG-CoA reductase inhibitor—a rate-limiting step in cholesterol biosynthesis ATP citrate lyase inhibitor—Upstream of HMG CoA reductase inhibition
LDLR Mediated	PCSK9 mAb (evolocumab, alirocumab) SiRNA that controls PCSK9 production (inclisiran)	Inhibits PCSK9-mediated LDL-R degradation Inhibits intracellular PCSK9 synthesis in hepatocytes by cleaving mRNA molecules encoding PCSK9
LDLR Independent LDL-C lowering	apoB ASO (mipomersan) MTTP inhibitor (lomitapide) ANGPTL3 inhibitors ANGPTL3 mAb (evinacumab) Anti-ANGPTL3 ASO (vupanorsen)	Pairs with apoB mRNA preventing its translation Inhibits MTTP—Blocks apoB loading onto TG, blocking VLDL assembly and secretion Blocks lipases, promotes VLDL remodeling, causes clearance of VLDL remnants via LDL-R independent uptake—Evinacumab as a mAb that blocks ANGPTL3 and vupanorsen by blocking ANGPTL3 synthesis

LDL-C low-density lipoprotein cholesterol, LDLR LDL receptor, *NPC1L1* Niemann-Pick C1-Like 1, *HMG CoA* hydroxymethylglutaryl-coenzyme A, *ATP* adenosine triphosphate, *PCSK9* proprotein convertase subtilisin/kexin type 9, *SiRNA* Small interfering RNA, *mRNA* messenger RNA, *ASO* anti-sense oligonucleotide, *apoB* apolipoprotein B100, *MTTP* microsomal triglyceride transfer protein, *TG* triglyceride, *VLDL* very-low-density lipoprotein, *ANGPTL3* Angiopoietin-like 3 protein, *mAb* monoclonal antibody

An FH treatment regimen should be tailored to achieve the recommended LDL-C levels. TLC and statin use are appropriate first line therapies, but additional medications may be necessary to achieve goal LDL-C levels. Additional therapeutic options for both HoFH and HeFH are described in Table 5.6. Lipid lowering therapies should also be considered in the setting of elevated non-HDL-C. Current recommendations suggest non-HDL-C be utilized in the setting of high triglycerides with a treatment goal of <145 mg/dL. Increasing evidence suggests that non-HDL-C and more specifically apoB are superior markers of risk stratification compared to LDL-C.

Several novel therapeutic agents are currently in development (Table 5.7). While data from adult clinical trials are informative, evidence demonstrating safety and efficiency in children, and ultimately FDA approval, will be needed prior to clinical use in youth less than 18 years-of-age. Nonetheless, newer therapeutic agents offer alternatives and have the potential of significantly helping reduce CVD risk and prevention of future ASCVD-related events in this population.

Clinical Vignettes

1. Patient 1 is an 11-year-old female seen for a routine health maintenance visit. She is active, enjoys playing competitive basketball, and easily keeps up with her peers. When at home, she is sedentary for ~2 h weekdays and ~4 h/day on weekends. She generally eats cereal for breakfast with 2% milk, her noon meal is provided by the school, and evening meals are usually consumed at home with her parents. Home meals commonly include vegetables. The family consumes juice occasionally but generally avoids sugar-sweetened beverages and sports drinks

   Her height is at the 68th, weight 76th· and BMI 78th percentile for age and sex. The physical examination is normal. The maternal grandfather has hypercholesterolemia and experienced a non-fatal MI at 53 years-of-age. He required two coronary artery stents. Her maternal uncle has hypercholesterolemia as well and began a statin in his 30s. Cholesterol levels are not known for the child's mother.

   The patient's lipid profile demonstrated: TC 292 mg/dL; HDL-C 58 mg/dL, LDL-C 213 mg/dL, TG 105 mg/dL. TSH, CMP, and urinalysis were all normal. Her Lp(a) was elevated at 120 mmol/L (expected <75 nmol/L). Genetic testing after pre-test counseling revealed a common pathologic LDL receptor mutation which was consistent with heterozygous FH. Cascade screening was recommended, which showed the mother and 1 of 3 siblings were also affected.

   Rosuvastatin 5 mg daily was recommended; following which the LDL-C decreased to 142 mg/dL. Since her LDL-C was not at goal (<100 mg/dL) despite adequate compliance, the rosuvastatin was increased to 10 mg/day. An LDL-C 3 months later was 128 mg/dL.
2. Patient 2 is a 14-year-old male referred by his primary care physician for dyslipidemia following a routine yearly physical examination. He is generally sedentary, with physical activities limited to walking between classes and an after-school job as a cashier in a local fast-food restaurant. A nutrition history reveals that he generally skips breakfast, eats lunch at school, and has his evening meal during work. In addition, he drinks approximately 24 ounces of sugar-sweetened beverages while at work. He denies cardiovascular symptoms. The family history is significant for a father who is obese with type 2 diabetes (T2D) and who, having experienced angina at 54 years-of-age, was required a coronary artery stent. A paternal uncle, who is not obese, also had coronary artery disease requiring a coronary artery bypass graft (CABG) at age 52. The patient's mother has no current medical problems. No additional family history is available

   The child's height is at the 48th percentile; weight and BMI >97th percentile. Prominent acanthosis nigricans and abdominal obesity were present on physical exam, which was otherwise unremarkable. A fasting lipid profile demonstrated: TC 264 mg/dL, HDL-C 28 mg/dL, and TG 418 mg/

dL. The LDL-C could not be calculated because TG were >400 mg/dL. Direct LDL-C was reported to be 178 mg/dL. His non-HDL-C was 236 mg/dL (markedly elevated). His hemoglobin $A1_C$ of 5.7% was consistent with "pre-diabetes" and ALT was mildly elevated at 47 U/L. Thyroid and renal function were normal.

Initial clinical findings were consistent with combined dyslipidemia of obesity (CDO). The family was provided counseling and encouraged to adopt changes consistent with a healthier lifestyle. Detailed instructions in heart healthy eating were provided by a registered dietician nutritionist. Following a 3-month trial of lifestyle modifications he lost 2 kg, however his weight and BMI percentile remained >99th percentile. A repeat lipid panel demonstrated TC 254 mg/dL, HDL-C 31 mg/dL, LDL-C 175 mg/dL, TG 240 mg/dL, non-HDL-C 223 mg/dL. Based upon his persistently elevated LDL-C and his family history, genetic testing was recommended which demonstrated a pathogenic variant in the LDL receptor. Thus, in addition to his obesity and insulin resistance/prediabetes, this child was found to have HeFH. The importance of therapeutic lifestyle changes, including weight management was reinforced and statin therapy initiated.

Hypocholesterolemia

Overview

Low levels of LDL-C or hypobetalipoproteinemia are defined as a total cholesterol (TC), LDL-C, and apoB <5th percentile for age and sex [9]. Depending upon its cause, a low level of LDL-C is generally associated with decreased risk of ASCVD. Low levels of LDL-C are most often seen in children who have moderate-to-severe hypertriglyceridemia, which primarily reflects impaired remodeling of TG-rich precursors of LDL. Secondary causes include malignancies, malabsorption syndromes, anemia, sepsis, chronic infections, and medication effects.

Genetic Variants

Children with loss of function variants in the genes for proprotein convertase subtilisin/kexin type 9 (PCSK9) and angiopoietin like protein 3 (ANGPTL3), have low but detectable LDL-C, without systemic involvement. Rare genetic conditions due to homozygous variants such as abetalipoproteinemia (ABL), homozygous familial

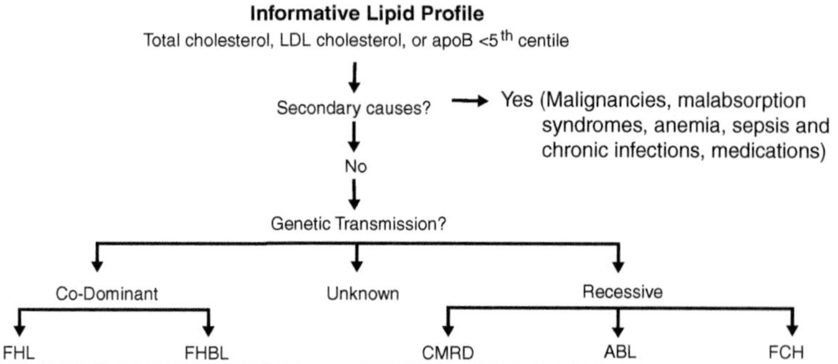

	FHL	FHBL	CMRD	ABL	FCH
Gene	*PCSK9*	*APOB*	*SAR1B*	*MTTP*	*ANGPTL3*
Heterozygous	Decreased CVD risk, otherwise no known clinical manifestations.	Generally asymptomatic, may develop fatty liver disease.	Generally asymptomatic	No clinical manifestations.	Generally asymptomatic
Homozygous*	Decreased CVD risk, otherwise no known clinical manifestations.	Variable, including FTT, steatorrhea, progressive neurologic and ophthalmologic abnormalities.	Variable, including FTT, steatorrhea, progressive neurologic abnormalities.	Variable: including FTT, steatorrhea, progressive neurologic and ophthalmologic abnormalities.	Generally asymptomatic

*Homozygous or compound heterozygous. FHL=Familial Hypolipoproteinemia; FHBL= Familial Hypobetalipoproteinemia; CMRD=Chylomicron Retention Disease; ABL=abetalipoproteinemia; FCH=Familial Combined Hypolipoproteinemia; FTT=Failure to

Modified from: Patrizia Tarugi and Maurizio Averna. Advances in Clinical Chemistry; Chapter 4. Hypobetalipoproteinemia: Genetics, biochemistry and clinical spectrum. Vol 54, 2011, Pg 100.

Fig. 5.2 Lipid test results

hypobetalipoproteinemia (FHBL), and chylomicron retention disease (CRD) manifest severe multisystem phenotypes characterized by the absence, or near absence, of LDL-C (Fig. 5.2). Clinical findings include steatorrhea, failure to thrive, and deficiency of fat-soluble vitamins, sometimes with retinopathy, coagulopathy, and progressive neurologic abnormalities. Most present in infancy or early childhood with one or more of these findings.

In contrast to homozygotes, children who have heterozygous gene variants are asymptomatic or less severely affected. Obligate heterozygotes for pathogenic microsomal triglyceride transfer (*MTTP*) mutations have normal lipid profiles and are generally asymptomatic. Individuals with heterozygous *APOB*-related FHBL have depressed, but not absent LDL-C. They may be identified through routine screening, cascade screening of an index case with homozygous FHBL or found coincidently during the evaluation of a child with a concomitant condition such as nonalcoholic fatty liver disease (NAFLD). Some children with heterozygous *APOB*-related FHBL appear to be at risk of developing fatty liver disease, although perhaps less severe than in NAFLD due to other causes. (Table 5.8).

Table 5.8 Initial evaluation and follow up of heterozygous hypobetalipoproteinemia. Adapted from (Jooho Lee & Robert A. Hegele. Abetalipoproteinemia and homozygous hypobetalipoproteinemia: a framework for diagnosis and management. J Inherit Metab Dis (2014) 37:333–339. https://doi.org/10.1007/s10545-013-9665-4; Levy E, Poinsot P, Spahis S. Chylomicron retention disease: genetics, biochemistry, and clinical spectrum. Curr Opin Lipidol. 2019 Apr;30(2):134–139. https://doi.org/10.1097/MOL.0000000000000578. PMID: 30640893; Peretti N, Sassolas A, Roy C, et al. Guidelines for the diagnosis and management of chylomicron retention disease based on a review of the literature and the experience of two centers. Orphanet Journal of Rare Diseases 2010;5:24, http://www.ojrd.com/content/5/1/24)

Variant	Inheritance	Initial evaluation	Follow-up	Clinical consequence
APOB (FHBL)	Autosomal dominant or co-dominant	Clinical judgement is recommended in those with depressed levels of apoB-containing lipoproteins. Obtaining initial clinical and laboratory evaluations may be reasonable	Clinical judgement is recommended in those with depressed levels of apoB-containing lipoproteins Regular monitoring of transaminases ± abdominal ultrasound may be reasonable, especially in those with conditions that may accelerate hepatic fibrosis, such as obesity, insulin resistance and diabetes mellitus	Mild, easily corrected fat-soluble vitamin deficiencies and hepatosteatosis may occur. More severe long-term hepatic complications have been reported but are rare
MTTP (ABL)	Autosomal recessive	Unnecessary	Unnecessary	Normal phenotype and lipid profile with no known clinical consequences. Heterozygous CRD may be identified by DNA analysis
SAR1B (CRD)	Autosomal recessive	Unnecessary	Unnecessary	Normal phenotype and lipid profile with no known clinical consequences. Heterozygous CRD may be identified by DNA analysis

ABL abetalipoproteinemia, *apoB* apolipoprotein B, *FHBL* familial hypobetalipoproteinemia, *CRD* chylomicron retention disease

The level of LDL-C, unfortunately, does not identify those at risk of fatty liver disease (i.e., heterozygous *APOB*-related FHBL) [10]. Furthermore, the plasma levels of LDL-C and apoB in heterozygous FHBL show wide inter-individual variability, even with the same variant and regardless of the underlying gene involved (*APOB* or *PCSK9*); which can confuse the clinical picture [11]. Missense variants in *PCSK9* are associated with hypocholesterolemia and possibly increased response to statin therapy [12].

This variability may be due to environmental factors, diet, or to interacting single gene or polygenic factors affecting secretion and catabolism of apoB-containing lipoproteins. An accurate diagnosis is important, however, since children with loss-of-function variants in *PCSK9*, as well as certain infections, malignancies, and medications have levels of LDL-C similar to those with heterozygous *APOB*-related FHBL, although they are not associated with fatty liver disease. In the absence of genetic testing, the decision to recommend further evaluation relies on a detailed, reliable, and informative family history, as well as the results of lipid testing and health histories of the first- and second-degree relatives [13].

In summary, the presence of a low LDL-C should be confirmed by a repeat lipid profile or a direct measurement of LDL-C. Secondary causes should be excluded, and genetic testing considered, the latter often informed by the family history.

Management

Children with a low level of cholesterol should be encouraged to adopt a heart-healthy lifestyle, including, a low-fat diet, daily exercise and maintain a healthy weight. Those with rare genetic conditions due to homozygous variants should be referred to an experienced multidisciplinary team for management (Table 5.8). Management and follow-up of children with heterozygous *APOB*-related FHBL poses a dilemma since some, but not all, are at risk of fatty liver disease. Since absorption of fat-soluble vitamins may be impaired, daily supplements should be encouraged. Monitoring of transaminases and an occasional liver ultrasound can be helpful in determining whether a child is developing fatty liver disease.

Conclusions

Abnormal LDL-C levels have broad clinical implications, ranging from cardioprotective when low to high risk of early ASCVD when elevated. Awareness and an increased level of suspicion, along with exclusion of secondary causes, selective use of additional biomarkers, a detailed family history, when available, and genetic testing assist clinicians in identifying the underlying mechanism of the LDL-C derangement. Such efforts significantly help reduce the morbidity and premature mortality associated with lifelong exposure to atherogenic lipoproteins. Use of cascade screening can extend the benefits of diagnosis and effective intervention to affected family members as well.

References

1. Expert Panel on Integrated Guidelines for Cardiovascular Health and Risk Reduction in Children and Adolescents; National Heart, Lung, and Blood Institute. Expert panel on integrated guidelines for cardiovascular health and risk reduction in children and adolescents: summary report. Pediatrics. 2011;128(Suppl 5):S215–56.
2. Benjamin EJ, Muntner P, Alonso A, Bittencourt MS, Callaway CW, Carson AP, et al. Heart disease and stroke Statistics-2019 update: a report from the American Heart Association. Circulation. 2019;139(10):e56–e528.
3. Feingold KR. Obesity and dyslipidemia. In: Feingold KR, Anawalt B, Boyce A, Chrousos G, de Herder WW, Dhatariya K, et al., editors. Endotext. South Dartmouth (MA): MDText.com, Inc; 2000.
4. Asselbergs FW, Guo Y, van Iperen EP, Sivapalaratnam S, Tragante V, Lanktree MB, et al. Large-scale gene-centric meta-analysis across 32 studies identifies multiple lipid loci. Am J Hum Genet. 2012;91(5):823–38.
5. Burns SF, Lee SJ, Arslanian SA. Surrogate lipid markers for small dense low-density lipoprotein particles in overweight youth. J Pediatr. 2012;161(6):991–6.
6. Cunniff C, Frias JL, Kaye C, Moeschler JB, Panny SR, Trotter TL, Hanson JW, Williams J, Moore CA, Lloyd-Puryear M, De la Cruz F, Cho S, Desposito F, Hoyme HE, Hall L. Molecular genetic testing in pediatric practice: a subject review. Committee on genetics. Pediatrics. 2000;106(6):1494–7.
7. de Ferranti SD, Steinberger J, Ameduri R, Baker A, Gooding H, Kelly AS, et al. Cardiovascular risk reduction in high-risk pediatric patients: a scientific statement from the American Heart Association. Circulation. 2019;139(13):e603–e34.
8. Vuorio A, Kuoppala J, Kovanen PT, Humphries SE, Tonstad S, Wiegman A, et al. Statins for children with familial hypercholesterolemia. Cochrane Database Syst Rev. 2019;2019(11):CD006401.
9. Hickman TB, Briefel RR, Carroll MD, Rifkind BM, Cleeman JI, Maurer KR, et al. Distributions and trends of serum lipid levels among United States children and adolescents ages 4-19 years: data from the third National Health and Nutrition Examination Survey. Prev Med. 1998;27(6):879–90.
10. Mouzaki M, Shah A, Arce-Clachar AC, Hardy J, Bramlage K, Xanthakos SA. Extremely low levels of low-density lipoprotein potentially suggestive of familial hypobetalipoproteinemia: a separate phenotype of NAFLD? J Clin Lipidol. 2019;13(3):425–31.
11. Cohen J, Pertsemlidis A, Kotowski IK, Graham R, Garcia CK, Hobbs HH. Low LDL cholesterol in individuals of African descent resulting from frequent nonsense mutations in PCSK9. Nat Genet. 2005;37(2):161–5.
12. Tarugi P, Averna M, Di Leo E, Cefalù AB, Noto D, Magnolo L, et al. Molecular diagnosis of hypobetalipoproteinemia: an ENID review. Atherosclerosis. 2007;195(2):e19–27.
13. Hartz J, Hegele RA, Wilson DP. Low LDL cholesterol-friend or foe? J Clin Lipidol. 2019;13(3):367–73.

Chapter 6
Therapies for Lowering Low-Density Lipoprotein Cholesterol

Nivedita Patni

Introduction

Cardiovascular disease (CVD) remains to be the leading cause of mortality in the United States. The current evidence supports that early identification and treatment of dyslipidemia in youth will significantly reduce clinical CVD risk in adult life. Etiology of hypercholesterolemia can be genetic, i.e. familial hypercholesterolemia (FH), polygenic hypercholesterolemia; or acquired secondary to conditions such as diabetes mellitus, nephrotic syndrome, and hypothyroidism. FH is an autosomal dominant disorder occurring in about 1 in 250 individuals, even more commonly in some ethnicities. Dyslipidemia due to obesity is commonly seen in childhood, and usually presents with mild elevation in total cholesterol (TC), variable low-density lipoprotein cholesterol (LDL-C), moderate-to-severe elevation in triglyceride (TG), and a low high-density cholesterol (HDL) level. In 2011, the National Heart Lung and Blood Institute (NHLBI), supported by American Academy of Pediatrics (AAP), issued Integrated Guidelines for Cardiovascular Health and Risk Reduction in Children and Adolescents [1]. The scientific statement issued in 2019 by American Heart Association described more detailed risk identification and treatment guidelines [2]. Lifestyle modifications with the "Cardiovascular Health Integrated Lifestyle diet" (CHILD—diet) and daily moderate-vigorous physical activity remain integral to the management of pediatric hypercholesterolemia; however, pharmacotherapy is essential in specific situations and has been evolving. Pharmacotherapy for the treatment of elevated LDL-C will be the focus of discussion in this chapter.

N. Patni (✉)
Department of Pediatrics, UT Southwestern Medical Center, Dallas, TX, USA
e-mail: nivedita.patni@utsouthwestern.edu

A. Ashraf, B. Sunil (eds.), *Pediatric Dyslipidemia*,
https://doi.org/10.1007/978-3-031-24113-0_6

Non-pharmacological Management

Lifestyle Changes

Per the NHLBI guidelines, fat intake in infants less than 12 months of age should not be restricted and breastfeeding should be encouraged. Between ages 1 and 2 years, as children transition from breast milk or formula, reduced fat milk (ranging from 2% milk to fat free milk) can be used based on the child's growth, appetite, and intake of other nutrient dense foods. For age > 1 year, the Expert Panel recommends following Cardiovascular Health Integrated Lifestyle Diet-1 (CHILD-1). If hypercholesterolemia persists after adequate compliance to CHILD-1 diet for 3 months, transition to LDL lowering CHILD-2 diet is recommended (Table 6.1). One hour per day of moderate-to-vigorous physical activity and <2 h per day of sedentary screen time are recommended for all patients over 5 years age. If the child is obese, nutrition therapy should include calorie restriction, and increased physical activity. Dietary interventions can reduce LDL-C by 10–13%.

Dietary Supplements

Water-soluble fiber psyllium and plant sterols may be added to CHILD-2 diet for children over 2 years. Psyllium at a dose 6 g/day for children 2–12 years and 12 g/day for children over 12 years can lower LDL-C and is well tolerated. Dietary supplement with approximately 2 g/day of plant sterols or stanols can lower LDL-C levels by 9–16%.

Table 6.1 Recommendations for dietary management of hypercholesterolemia (Adapted from National Heart, Blood and Lung Institute Expert Panel on Integrated Guidelines for Cardiovascular Health and Risk Reduction in Children and Adolescents [1])

CHILD-1 diet	Total fat 30% of daily kcal Saturated fat 8–10% of daily kcal Monounsaturated and polyunsaturated fat up to 20% of daily kcal Cholesterol less than 300 mg/day[a] Avoid trans fat
Child-2 LDL-C diet	Total fat 25–30% of daily kcal Saturated fat ≤7% of daily kcal Monounsaturated and polyunsaturated fat up to 10% of daily kcal Cholesterol 200 mg/day[a] Avoid trans fat

CHILD Cardiovascular Health Integrated Lifestyle Diet
[a]Dietary Guidelines for Americans (2015–2020) by US Departments of Health and Human Services (DHHS) and Agriculture (USDA) did not specify limiting consumption of dietary cholesterol because of inadequate evidence

Pharmacological Management

When to Start Pharmacological Therapy

Treatment for children with elevated LDL-C is based on assessment of lipid levels and associated risk for atherosclerotic coronary artery pathology as detailed in Table 6.2. Decisions regarding initiation of drug therapy should be based on the average of results from at least two fasting lipid panels obtained at minimum of 2 weeks but no more than 3 months apart. Positive family history includes premature CVD in first or second degree relative (myocardial infarction, stroke, angina, coronary artery bypass, stent, angioplasty, or sudden cardiac death before age 55 year in a male or before age 65 year in a female) or a known diagnosis of FH, tendon xanthoma, or total cholesterol >290 mg/dL. The guidelines for pharmacotherapy are detailed in Table 6.2.

Pharmacologic Therapy Goals

The minimum goal of LDL-C lowering therapy in childhood and adolescence is to achieve LDL-C <130 mg/dL (95th percentile) (Table 6.2). A lower LDL-C of <100 mg/dL is advised for patients with high-risk categories as described in Table 6.2.

HMG-CoA Reductase Inhibitors (Statins)

The statins are the first line of pharmacologic therapy to treat children with hypercholesterolemia persistent after diet and lifestyle changes. Large-scale evidence from randomized trials have shown that statin therapy reduces the risk of major vascular events during each year it continues to be taken, thus larger absolute benefits accumulate with prolonged therapy, which persist long term. Arterial wall changes begin to occur in childhood in patients with FH. Statin therapy initiation during childhood in these patients have shown to slow down the progression of carotid intima-media thickness [3] and reduces the risk of CVD [4]. Safety and efficacy of statin use in children has been established by several randomized double-blind placebo-controlled trials and meta-analysis studies [5]. A recent 20-year follow-up study of statin therapy in 214 children with familial hypercholesterolemia showed statin therapy decreased LDL-C levels by 32% from baseline level. Information on cardiovascular events for 203 patients and 156 parents with familial hypercholesterolemia showed that the cumulative CVD-free survival at 39 years of age was 99% among patients with familial hypercholesterolemia who started statin therapy during childhood and was 74% among their affected parents (hazard ratio

Table 6.2 Risk categorization and treatment decision-making in patients with hypercholesterolemia (Adapted from Expert Panel on Integrated Guidelines for Cardiovascular Health and Risk Reduction in Children and Adolescents, National Heart, Lung, and Blood Institute, 2011 [1]; and Cardiovascular risk reduction in high-risk pediatric patients: A scientific statement from the American Heart Association, 2019 [2])

	High risk	Moderate risk	At risk
Risk factors	Homozygous FH Type 1 or type 2 diabetes mellitus Kawasaki disease with persistent coronary aneurysms End-stage renal disease Solid-organ transplant vasculopathy Childhood cancer survivor after stem cell transplantation Multiple comorbidities—Any moderate-risk condition plus ≥2 additional risk enhancers	Severe obesity (BMI ≥99th percentile or ≥35 kg/m^2) Confirmed hypertension (BP >95th percentile or ≥130/80 mmHg on three separate occasions) Childhood cancer survivor with exposure to chest irradiation Chronic kidney disease Heterozygous FH Kawasaki disease with regressed coronary aneurysms Multiple risk factors—≥3 risk enhancers	Obesity (BMI ≥95th to <99th percentile) Insulin resistance with comorbidities (e.g., NAFLD, PCOS) Current smoker or significant exposure to second-hand smoke White-coat hypertension Chronic inflammatory disease (e.g., SLE, systemic JIA) HIV infection Childhood cancer survivor with cardiotoxic chemotherapy only Adolescent depressive and bipolar disorders Congenital heart disease involving (1) obstructive lesions of the left ventricle and aorta; (2) cyanotic congenital heart defects leading to Eisenmenger syndrome; and (3) congenital coronary artery anomalies, in isolation or in association with other congenital defects. Biomarkers: • Elevated Lp(a) • Elevated apolipoprotein B
LDL-C threshold	≥130 mg/dL	≥160 mg/dL	≥160 mg/dL
Treatment	Initiate statin and lifestyle change	Lifestyle change for 3 months	Lifestyle change for 6 months
		Statin if LDL-C above goal	Statin if LDL-C above goal
LDL-C treatment goal	<100 mg/dL	<130 mg/dL	<130 mg/dL

FH familial hypercholesterolemia, *BMI* body mass index, *BP* blood pressure, *NAFLD* nonalcoholic fatty liver disease, *PCOS* polycystic ovary syndrome, *CVD* cardiovascular disease, *TC* total cholesterol, *SLE* systemic lupus erythematosus, *JIA* juvenile idiopathic arthritis, *HCM* hypertrophic cardiomyopathy, *TGA* transposition of the great arteries

with adjustment for sex and smoking status, 11.8; 95% CI, 3.0–107.0). Mean progression of carotid intima–media thickness of 184 patients was compared to their unaffected siblings. The rate of progression in mean carotid intima–media thickness was 0.0056 mm (95% CI, 0.0051–0.0061) per year in the patients compared to 0.0057 mm (95% CI, 0.0050–0.0065) per year in their unaffected siblings (mean difference adjusted for sex, −0.0001 mm per year; 95% CI, −0.0010–0.0008) [6].

Table 6.3 FDA-approved pediatric dosing, effect of LDL reduction (pediatric data), and properties of statin drug therapy [7]

Statin	Dose range (mg/day)	Effect on LDL reduction	Lipophilicity	CYP substrate
Pitavastatin	2–4	30–38%	Lipophilic	2C9
Pravastatin	20–40	24–33%	Hydrophilic	Sulfation
Rosuvastatin	5–20	38–50%	Hydrophilic	2C9
Atorvastatin	10–20	38–44%	Lipophilic	3A4
Fluvastatin	20–80	23–34%	Lipophilic	2C9
Lovastatin	10–40	17–36%	Lipophilic	3A4
Simvastatin	5–40	25–41%	Lipophilic	3A4

Statins decrease the hepatic synthesis of cholesterol by competitive inhibition of HMG-CoA reductase, which is the rate-limiting step in cholesterol biosynthesis. Decrease in intrahepatic cholesterol levels upregulates the LDL-C receptor expression in the liver, causing increased clearance of apolipoprotein-B containing lipoproteins (LDL and VLDL), causing decrease of plasma total cholesterol and LDL-C levels. In the USA, pitavastatin, pravastatin, and rosuvastatin are FDA (U.S. Food and Drug Administration) approved for children 8 years and older; and atorvastatin, fluvastatin, lovastatin, and simvastatin are approved for children 10 years and older. Rosuvastatin and Atorvastatin have been approved from 6 years age in Europe and Australia, respectively. The recommended dosing range are detailed in Table 6.3.

The statins should be started at the lowest dose after getting baseline measurements of fasting lipid profile, aspartate aminotransferase, alanine aminotransferase, and creatine kinase. Physician should perform extensive counseling to patients and family members regarding potential adverse events. Statins have been contraindicated in pregnancy, and females should be informed about the need to avoid pregnancy and breastfeeding while using statins, and to stop them 3 months before pregnancy; however, FDA has recently requested to remove the strongest warning against using statins during pregnancy. A fasting lipid profile, aspartate aminotransferase, alanine aminotransferase, and creatine kinase should be repeated 4 and 8 weeks after initiation of therapy, and then every 3–6 months. Statins should be discontinued if the liver enzymes are above three times the upper limit of normal, creatinine kinase is above 10 times the upper limit of normal, or patient develops adverse effects to therapy [1].

Statins are usually very well tolerated in children and have excellent safety profile. A meta-analysis of six randomized, double-blind, placebo-controlled trials evaluating statin therapy in children, aged 8–18 years, with heterozygous familial hypercholesterolemia (HeFH) showed no statistically significant differences in the occurrence of adverse events (relative risk (RR) 0.99; 95% CI, 0.79–1.25, 5]. There was a minimal difference in growth, in favor of the statin group (0.33 cm; 95% CI, 0.03–0.63 cm) in four studies which reported data on height [5]. Three studies reported sexual development, showing no significant difference between the two groups (RR of advancing to next Tanner stage classification was 0.96; 95% CI, 0.79–1.17) [5]. Asymptomatic elevation of (RR of CK ≥10 upper limit of normal

(ULN) 1.38; 95% CI, 0.18–10.82), and liver enzymes (RR of ≥3 times the ULN for aspartate aminotransferase (AST) 0.98; 95% CI, 0.23–4.26, and for alanine transaminase (ALT) 2.03; 95% CI, 0.24–16.95) were not statistically significant [5]. In adults, 1/500 to 1/1000 patients may develop myositis on a statin, which can lead to life-threatening rhabdomyolysis; however, it has not been reported in children. Even in adults, rhabdomyolysis is extremely rare, and the recommendations are to check CK in the case of severe statin-associated muscle symptoms and in the presence of objective muscle weakness [7]. FDA recommends measuring baseline AST and ALT in adults and repeat if there are signs or symptoms suggesting hepatotoxicity [7]. Atorvastatin, lovastatin, and simvastatin are metabolized by the CYP3A4 isozyme of the cytochrome P450 microsomal enzyme system (Table 6.3), and therefore can have drug interactions with other agents metabolized by CYP3A4, including cyclosporine, erythromycin, verapamil, HIV protease inhibitors, sertraline, and gemfibrozil. Larger intake of grapefruit juice with these agents can also inhibit CYP3A4.

Bile Acid Sequestrants

Bile acid sequestrants (BAS) or bile acid-binding resins were the only class of medications recommended by NCEP Pediatric Panel Report in 1992. They bind the bile acids in the intestine interrupting their enterohepatic circulation, hence stimulating the conversion of cholesterol to bile acids in the liver. This results in lowering of the hepatic cholesterol level and inducing LDL receptors, causing increased clearance of LDL-C. They have additive LDL-cholesterol-lowering effects when combined with statin therapy; however, their side effects and tolerability make their use clinically challenging. Cholestyramine (8 g/day) can lower LDL-C by approximately 15% compared to placebo in patients with familial hypercholesterolemia; however, compliance is a challenge due to unpalatability and gastrointestinal side effects. Colestipol granules (10 g/day) or tablets (2–12 g/day) have shown to decrease LDL-C by 20%; however, adherence is a challenge with these as well due to similar reasons as cholestyramine. Besides causing significant gastrointestinal side effects, they have also been shown to decrease serum folate levels, and 25-hydroxyvitamin D deficiency. Colesevelam (3.75 g/day) has been shown to lower LDL-C by 14% and has a better tolerability than cholestyramine. The tablets are also smaller in size and easier to administer. It is FDA approved for children ≥10 years with heterozygous hypercholesterolemia [8].

Cholesterol Absorption Inhibitors (Ezetimibe)

Ezetimibe inhibits the NPC1L1 (Niemann-Pick C1 Like Intracellular Cholesterol Transporter 1) protein transporter, blocking the absorption of dietary and biliary cholesterol. This causes upregulation of LDL-receptor expression and increased clearance of LDL-C from plasma. Ezetimibe (10 mg/day) can lower LDL-C by

28–30% when used alone [9, 10] or combined with a statin [11]. Clinical trials have shown safety and efficacy of ezetimibe in children as young as 5 years age [9, 10]. A multi-center, randomized, double blinded, placebo-controlled study of 248 patients, age 10–17 years, showed that co-administration of ezetimibe with simvastatin caused 54% reduction in LDL-C compared to 34% by simvastatin monotherapy. The authors also showed safety and tolerability of this combination therapy for up to 53 weeks [11]. Ezetimibe along with elimination of plant sterols is the mainstay of therapy for patients with sitosterolemia [12].

PCSK9 Inhibitors

PCSK9 inhibitors target human proprotein convertase subtilisin/kexin type 9 (PCSK9) and prevent it from degrading low-density lipoprotein receptor (LDLR). Its effects in lowering LDL-C have shown to be additive, not synergistic, with statin therapy. Evolocumab is a fully human monoclonal antibody directed against PCSK9, which was approved to reduce LDL-C in adults in 2015. A recent 24-week, randomized, double-blind, placebo-controlled trial of monthly evolocumab (420 mg) in 157 pediatric patients (age range 10–17 years) with heterozygous familial hypercholesterolemia showed reduction of LDL-C by 38.3% (95% CI, −45.5–−31.1; $p < 0.0001$) from baseline compared to placebo [13]. The most common adverse events were nasopharyngitis, headache, oropharyngeal pain, influenza, upper respiratory tract infection, and gastroenteritis; however, the incidence of adverse events was similar in the evolocumab and the placebo group [13]. In September 2021, the FDA approved evolocumab for the treatment of pediatric patients aged 10 years and older with heterozygous familial hypercholesterolemia (HeFH) as an adjunct to diet and other LDL-C lowering therapies. Alirocumab is also a fully human monoclonal antibody which binds PCSK9 with high affinity but is not FDA approved for the pediatric population at the time of writing this chapter.

Fibrates

Fibrates (Fibric acid derivatives) activate the peroxisome proliferator-activated receptor alpha (PPAR alpha), which upregulates the gene for LPL causing lipolysis and reduction of triglyceride. Fibrates also upregulate the gene for apo A-I and apo A-II, which increases HDL-C production and enhances reverse cholesterol transport. They can induce structural change in LDL-C receptors as well and can decrease LDL-C by about 8%. Fibrates are not FDA approved for use in children and they are usually reserved for youth with severe fasting hypertriglyceridemia associated with risk of pancreatitis but are ineffective in children with very low or absent LPL [1]. In adults, fibrate-statin combinations are used in patients with mixed dyslipidemia; however, fibric acid derivatives, particularly gemfibrozil, increase the incidence of adverse events such as rhabdomyolysis, when used with statins.

Niacin

Niacin (Nicotinic acid) inhibits hepatic diglycerol acyltransferase2 (DGAT2) and the release of free fatty acids from adipose tissue, decreasing VLDL and LDL cholesterol production and HDL cholesterol degradation. Long term niacin use in adults was associated with hyperglycemia and new onset type 2 diabetes. Based on systematic reviews there are no positive cardiovascular risk benefits for niacin. One retrospective review showed that niacin (>1000 mg/day) reduced LDL-C by 30% in 21 children (age 4–14 years); however 76% children experienced adverse effects, and 38% discontinued therapy due to flushing, abdominal pain, vomiting, headache, or elevated serum aminotransferase levels. It is not FDA approved for use in the pediatric population. Due to the high prevalence of adverse effects, use of niacin is not recommended in children.

Omega-3 Fish Oils

Omega-3 fish oils (ω-3 fatty acids) enriched in eicosapentaenoic acid (EPA) and docosahexaenoic acid (DHA) reduce apo-C III plasma levels via the PPARα pathway and decrease hepatic fatty acid and triglycerides synthesis while augmenting fatty acid degradation/oxidation: causing overall reduction in VLDL cholesterol release. Both EPA and DHA lower triglycerides and raises HDL cholesterol; however, DHA has been shown to increase mean LDL cholesterol from a baseline of 0.2–10.9%. The prescription formulations of ω-3 fatty acids are not yet FDA approved for children.

Treatment Modalities for Specific Conditions

1. **Lipoprotein(a) [Lp(a)]:** Lp(a) is a lipid-rich apo B-containing lipoprotein that has pro-atherogenic, pro-thrombotic, pro-inflammatory, and pro-oxidative properties and has been associated with poor cardiovascular prognosis. Early and lifelong implementation of a heart-healthy lifestyle is the key treatment strategy and statins have not been shown to lower Lp(a) levels. PCSK9 inhibitors can significantly reduce Lp(a) levels, and patients with higher baseline Lp(a) levels have higher absolute reductions in Lp(a) levels. Lipid apheresis has been successfully used in youth with high Lp(a) and recurrent ischemic stroke [14].
2. **Sitosterolemia**: Sitosterolemia is an autosomal recessive disorder caused by pathogenic biallelic variants in *ABCG5* or *ABCG8*, which result in increased intestinal absorption and decreased biliary excretion of sterols. Dietary restriction of non-cholesterol sterols and ezetimibe are the mainstay of therapy [12]. Bile acid sequestrants may be considered; however, sitosterolemic patients do not respond to statins.

3. **Lysosomal acid lipase deficiency (LAL-D):** LAL-D is an autosomal recessive disorder caused by homozygous or compound heterozygous mutations in *LIPA*. Deficiency of LAL results in diminished hydrolysis of cholesteryl esters and triglycerides, trapping the cholesterol esters and triglycerides within the lysosomes in liver and spleen, along with other organs. Kanuma® (sebelipase alfa), a recombinant human lysosomal acid lipase, is approved by the FDA to treat LAL-D.
4. **Cerebrotendinous Xanthomatosis (CTX):** CTX is an autosomal-recessive disorder caused by homozygous or compound heterozygous mutation in the *CYP27A1*. Patients with CTX lack mitochondrial sterol 27-hydroxylase, which prevents the synthesis of chenodeoxycholic acid (CDCA) and cholic acid, and abnormal deposition of cholestanol and cholesterol in multiple tissues presenting with skin xanthomas, early cataracts and chronic diarrhea and jaundice in children. A sterol profile (including cholestanol by Gas Chromatography-Mass Spectrometry is currently available at Mayo Clinic labs. Early initiation of chenodeoxycholic acid (250 mg given three times daily for adults and 15 mg/kg/d for children) is the treatment of choice for neurological and non-neurological symptoms [15].
5. **Homozygous Familial Hypercholesterolemia (HoFH):** HoFH is caused by pathogenic variants in both LDL receptor (*LDLR*) alleles (~ 90% patients), apolipoprotein B (*APOB*), proprotein convertase subtilisin/kexin type 9 (*PCSK9*) or, rarely, the LDL receptor adaptor protein 1 (*LDLRAP1*) (autosomal recessive hypercholesterolemia - ARH). If untreated, these patients can have fatal coronary insufficiency or myocardial infarction before the age of 20. Statins, ezetimibe, and bile acid sequestrants have lesser LDL-C-lowering effect in HoFH because their mechanism of actions depend on some LDL receptor functionality to be fully effective. However, *Rosuvastatin* has been shown to reduce LDL-C by ~22% in LDLR defective mutations, and ~ 13% reduction in LDL-C in LDLR negative mutations [16]. The Trial Evaluating PCSK9 antibody in Subjects With LDL Receptor (TESLA) study in 12 patients, age 14 to 54 years, showed reductions of 16.5% (range, 5.2%−−43.6%; $P = 0.0781$) and 13.9% (range, 39.9%−−43.3%; $P = 0.1484$) with *evolocumab* 420 mg every 4 weeks and every 2 weeks, respectively, over 12 weeks duration [17]. The two patients carrying negative LDLR mutations did not have any LDL-C reduction, however, the six subjects carrying defective LDLR mutations had a significant decrease of LDL-C (−19% and −26%) with 4- and 2-week dosing, respectively [17]. *Mipomersen* (200 mg weekly), an antisense inhibitor of apoB synthesis, given subcutaneously, can reduce LDL-C by 42% by 26 weeks; however injection site reactions, flu like symptoms and elevated liver enzymes are common [18]. A 24 week, double-blind, placebo-controlled, phase 3 trial of *Evinacumab* (monoclonal antibody against ANGPTL3) in 65 patients with HoFH showed a relative reduction from baseline of 47.1% in the LDL-C in the study group, compared with an increase of 1.9% in the placebo group (95% CI, −65.0 to −33.1; $P < 0.001$). The study had one adolescent patient (age 12–18) in each group, and the medication was administered at dose of 15 mg/kg intravenously every 4 weeks [19]. *Lomitapide*,

an oral inhibitor of the microsomal triglyceride transfer protein, has shown to reduce LDL-C levels by 50% in adults with HoFH, effects sustained for up to 78 weeks [20]. However, Lomitapide is not approved for children in the USA. *Lipoprotein apheresis* is removal of lipoproteins from the circulation and can be considered by 5 years of age in patients with HoFH, and has been shown to reduce LDL-C by more than 60% [21]. Lipoprotein apheresis is carried out weekly or biweekly in HoFH patients if LDL targets are not achieved with maximal combined statin plus combination therapy [22]. In the U SA, HELP (Heparin-induced extracorporeal LDL precipitation) and dextran sulfate adsorption (Liposorber) are approved by the FDA [21]. *Liver transplantation* has been described as treatment, which lowers LDL-C by correcting the molecular defect underlying the disease [23, 24].

Conclusion

Non-pharmacologic and pharmacologic therapy for LDL-C lowering have greatly expanded in last few decades. Lifestyle modifications with the "CHILD—diet" and daily moderate-vigorous physical activity remain essential for pediatric hypercholesterolemia management; however, the pharmacotherapy has been evolving. Statin (HMG-CoA reductase inhibitors) is the first-line pharmacologic treatment for children and adolescents with severe hypercholesterolemia persistent despite the diet and exercise interventions. Bile acid sequestrants, ezetimibe, and PCSK9 inhibitor (evolocumab) have been shown to be efficacious and safe for children with hypercholesterolemia. In the last decade, there has been a significant increase in data available on the use of cholesterol lowering medications in children and adolescents; however, long-term study data are still not available and continues to be an active focus of research.

References

1. Expert Panel on Integrated Guidelines for Cardiovascular Health and Risk Reduction in Children and Adolescents; National Heart, Lung, and Blood Institute. Expert panel on integrated guidelines for cardiovascular health and risk reduction in children and adolescents: summary report. Pediatrics. 2011;128(Suppl 5):S213–56.
2. de Ferranti SD, et al. Cardiovascular risk reduction in high-risk pediatric patients: a scientific statement from the American Heart Association. Circulation. 2019;139(13):e603–34.
3. Wiegman A, et al. European atherosclerosis society consensus panel. Familial hypercholesterolaemia in children and adolescents: gaining decades of life by optimizing detection and treatment. Eur Heart J. 2015;36(36):2425–37.
4. Wiegman A. Lipid screening, action, and follow-up in children and adolescents. Curr Cardiol Rep. 2018;20(9):80.
5. Avis HJ, et al. A systematic review and meta-analysis of statin therapy in children with familial hypercholesterolemia. Arterioscler Thromb Vasc Biol. 2007;27(8):1803–10.

6. Luirink IK, et al. 20-year follow-up of statins in children with familial hypercholesterolemia. N Engl J Med. 2019;381:1547.
7. Grundy SM, et al. 2018 AHA/ACC/AACVPR/AAPA/ABC/ACPM/ADA/AGS/APhA/ASPC/NLA/PCNA guideline on the management of blood cholesterol: executive summary: a report of the American College of Cardiology/American Heart Association task force on clinical practice guidelines. J Am Coll Cardiol. 2019;73(24):3168–209.
8. Stein EA, et al. Colesevelam hydrochloride: efficacy and safety in pediatric subjects with heterozygous familial hypercholesterolemia. J Pediatr. 2010;156(2):231–6 e1–3.
9. Yeste D, et al. Ezetimibe as monotherapy in the treatment of hypercholesterolemia in children and adolescents. J Pediatr Endocrinol Metab. 2009;22(6):487–92.
10. Clauss S, et al. Ezetimibe treatment of pediatric patients with hypercholesterolemia. J Pediatr. 2009;154(6):869–72.
11. van der Graaf A, et al. Efficacy and safety of coadministration of ezetimibe and simvastatin in adolescents with heterozygous familial hypercholesterolemia. J Am Coll Cardiol. 2008;52(17):1421–9.
12. Salen G, et al. Ezetimibe effectively reduces plasma plant sterols in patients with sitosterolemia. Circulation. 2004;109(8):966–71.
13. Santos RD, et al. Evolocumab in pediatric heterozygous familial hypercholesterolemia. N Engl J Med. 2020;383(14):1317–27.
14. Wilson DP, Koschinsky ML, Moriarty PM. Expert position statements: comparison of recommendations for the care of adults and youth with elevated lipoprotein(a). Curr Opin Endocrinol Diabetes Obes. 2021;28(2):159–73.
15. Stelten BM, et al. Long-term treatment effect in cerebrotendinous xanthomatosis depends on age at treatment start. Neurology. 2019;92(2):e83–95.
16. Stein EA, et al. Efficacy of Rosuvastatin in children with homozygous familial hypercholesterolemia and association with underlying genetic mutations. J Am Coll Cardiol. 2017;70(9):1162–70.
17. Stein EA, et al. Effect of the proprotein convertase subtilisin/kexin 9 monoclonal antibody, AMG 145, in homozygous familial hypercholesterolemia. Circulation. 2013;128(19):2113–20.
18. Raal FJ, et al. Pediatric experience with mipomersen as adjunctive therapy for homozygous familial hypercholesterolemia. J Clin Lipidol. 2016;10(4):860–9.
19. Raal FJ, et al. Evinacumab for homozygous familial hypercholesterolemia. N Engl J Med. 2020;383(8):711–20.
20. Perry CM. Lomitapide: a review of its use in adults with homozygous familial hypercholesterolemia. Am J Cardiovasc Drugs. 2013;13(4):285–96.
21. Moriarty PM, Hemphill L. Lipoprotein apheresis. Endocrinol Metab Clin N Am. 2016;45(1):39–54.
22. Harada-Shiba M, et al. Guidance for pediatric familial hypercholesterolemia 2017. J Atheroscler Thromb. 2018;25(6):539–53.
23. Cuchel M, et al. Homozygous familial hypercholesterolaemia: new insights and guidance for clinicians to improve detection and clinical management. A position paper from the consensus panel on familial hypercholesterolaemia of the European Atherosclerosis Society. Eur Heart J. 2014;35(32):2146–57.
24. Gidding SS, et al. The agenda for familial hypercholesterolemia: a scientific statement from the American Heart Association. Circulation. 2015;132(22):2167–92.

Chapter 7
Combined Dyslipidemia

Rae-Ellen W. Kavey

Combined Dyslipidemia

Definition

The combination of high triglyceride (TG) levels with low high-density lipoprotein cholesterol (HDL-C) is the most common abnormal lipid pattern in childhood and adolescence. The most recent guidelines on lipid management in childhood from the National Heart, Lung, and Blood Institute (NHLBI) define combined dyslipidemia (CD) based on normal lipid profile results as shown in Table 7.1 [1]. A diagnosis of CD requires that the average of a least two fasting measurements of TG are above the 95th percentile, plus HDL-C at or below the fifth percentile. In the typical lipid profile of a child or adolescent with CD, TG levels are between 150 and 400 mg/dL and HDL-C is <40 mg/dL [2]. Total cholesterol (TC) and low-density lipoprotein cholesterol (LDL-C) levels may also be mildly elevated, but this is not required for CD diagnosis.

Pathophysiology

TGs, also known as triacylglycerols, are esters derived from glycerol and three fatty acids. They are core components of all lipoproteins, especially the apolipoprotein-B48 (apoB 48) containing chylomicrons produced in the intestine in response to dietary fat, and apo B 100 containing very-low-density lipoproteins (VLDL) produced in the liver. TGs are the main constituents of body fat and are important in

---

R.-E. W. Kavey (✉)
University of Rochester Medical Center, Rochester, NY, USA

A. Ashraf, B. Sunil (eds.), *Pediatric Dyslipidemia*,
https://doi.org/10.1007/978-3-031-24113-0_7

Table 7.1 Acceptable, borderline, and high plasma lipid, lipoprotein, and apolipoprotein concentrations (mg/dL) for children and adolescents*

Category	Acceptable	Borderline high	High*
TC	<170	170–199	≥200
LDL-C	<110	110–129	≥130
Non-HDL-C	<120	120–144	≥145
ApoB	<90	90–109	≥110
TG			
0–9 years	<75	75–99	≥100
10–19 years	<90	90–129	≥130
Category	**Acceptable**	**Borderline high**	**Low***
HDL-C	>45	40–45	<40
ApoA-I	>120	115–120	<115

NOTE: Values given are in mg/dL; to convert to SI units, divide the results for TC, LDL-C, HDL-C and non-HDL-C by 38.6; for TG, divide by 88.6

*The cut points for high and borderline high represent the 95th and 75th percentiles, respectively. Low cut points for HDL-C and apoA-I represent approximately the 10th percentile

energy metabolism, hydrolyzed to provide free fatty acids for energy metabolism, with the excess stored in adipose tissue. Mild-to-moderate TG elevations primarily represent accumulation of VLDL and remnant lipoprotein particles, while excess chylomicrons, accompanied by excess VLDL and remnant lipoproteins, are predominant in severe HTG [3]. In the typical lipid profile of a child or adolescent with CD, TG elevation is mild to moderate. From National Health and Nutrition Examination Survey (NHANES) data, severe TG concentrations of >500 mg/dL are rare, accounting for <0.2% of the HTG cases in children, but if sustained should prompt consideration of an associated genetic abnormality [3].

Extreme TG levels, above 1000 mg/dL, are exceedingly rare and are associated with significant risk of acute pancreatitis. Elevation to this level strongly suggests an underlying genetic trait, either a mutation in the lipoprotein lipase (LPL) complex (LPL, APOC2, APOA5, LMF1, GPIHBP1), termed the familial chylomicronemia syndrome (FCS), or the co-existence of minor genetic and secondary forms of HTG, termed the multifactorial chylomicronemia syndrome. Environmental factors can play an important role in phenotype expression in both settings. The exact mechanism by which hypertriglyceridemia causes pancreatitis is not clearly understood, with most accepted theories based on animal models which describe metabolism of excessive TGs by lipoprotein lipase into free fatty acids, leading to pancreatic cell injury and ischemia. Confirmed TG levels above 1000 mg/dL identify a child who requires genetic evaluation and specific TG management to minimize the risk for pancreatitis [3].

The terminology describing combined dyslipidemia also includes "mixed dyslipidemia" and "atherogenic dyslipidemia," with combined dyslipidemia used most commonly in pediatrics. There is overlap in the lipid phenotype between CD and the classic definition of familial combined hyperlipidemia

(FCHL) which was originally considered to be a genetically discrete entity. However, current evidence suggests that FCHL is a multigenic dyslipidemia with variable expression in different pedigrees. There is well-established familial aggregation of the combined dyslipidemia phenotype in pediatric and adult studies, beyond the historic studies of FCHL. Emerging evidence from gene sequencing studies suggests that minor variants in the genes controlling TG metabolism may be important factors in the expression of hypertriglyceridemia and combined dyslipidemia [2].

Prevalence

In youth, CD occurs almost exclusively with obesity and with the sustained high prevalence of obesity, CD is also highly prevalent. Results from the NHANES for 2017–2018 show that 19.3% of US children and adolescents aged 2–19 years have obesity, including 6.1% with severe obesity [4]. In cross-sectional data from multiple populations, 30–60% of obese youth have CD with the prevalence increasing as obesity severity increases.

CD is strongly associated with a complex of related cardiometabolic factors including visceral adiposity, insulin resistance (IR)/type 2 diabetes (T2DM), non-alcoholic fatty liver disease (NAFLD), and the metabolic syndrome (MetS). In susceptible individuals with an underlying racial/ethnic/familial/genetic predisposition, excessive weight gain occurs disproportionately as visceral fat (VAT). Waist circumference (WC) is an effective measure of VAT/ abdominal obesity in youth, with measures above the 90th percentile for age/sex strongly predicting CD with high TGs and reduced HDL-C [2].

Obesity correlates with hyperinsulinemia in children, adolescents and adults and IR is associated with abdominal obesity and CD. During puberty, IR is physiologic with an average 50% decrease in insulin sensitivity; the pattern of IR is exaggerated in obese adolescents and persists after puberty. IR and CD are seen only in obese subjects and the dyslipidemia correlates with the degree of IR. Progression from IR to impaired fasting glucose to T2DM has been documented in youth, especially where there is a family history of diabetes. T2DM is increasingly common in obese adolescents with prevalence doubling from 0.34 per 1000 youths to 0.67 per 1000 youths between 2001 and 2017 [5].

CD is also strongly linked with non-alcoholic fatty liver disease (NAFLD), defined as hepatic fat infiltration in >5% of hepatocytes without evidence of hepatocellular injury on liver biopsy. NAFLD is highly correlated with obesity, especially abdominal obesity, affecting at least 38% of obese adolescents in autopsy series and ~ 50% in epidemiologic surveys. In more than half of NAFLD subjects, the CD pattern is present on standard lipid profile and with nuclear magnetic resonance (NMR) analysis. In children and adolescents, NAFLD is associated with atherosclerosis at autopsy and with ultrasound vascular markers of atherosclerosis.

CD, visceral adiposity, IR and NAFLD are each associated with MetS, a long-established high-risk constellation for atherosclerotic disease. In the USA, MetS is reported in 23% of adults, including almost 7% of 20–30-year-olds. In childhood, the MetS cluster was found in 29% of obese adolescents compared with 0.1% of those with a normal BMI. Presence of the MetS cluster at a mean age of 12 years is an independent predictor of adult cardiovascular disease (CVD) 25 years later [6].

In summary, CD is strongly associated with multiple, interrelated cardiometabolic factors. When visceral adiposity develops in children and adolescents with an underlying metabolic/genetic/familial predisposition, a cascade of pathophysiologic reactions occurs, resulting in CD, IR/T2DM, and NAFLD and when combined MetS. These prevalent combinations are powerful predictors of cardiometabolic risk.

Atherogenicity

Advanced lipid profile analysis by NMR spectroscopy reveals that at the lipid subpopulation level, the CD pattern is represented as increased small, dense LDL (sdLDL-C) and LDL particle number. High LDL particle number and sdLDL-C have each been shown to predict clinical CVD with elevated sdLDL-C shown to be the most atherogenic lipoprotein parameter in the prospective Framingham Offspring Study [7].

An important initiating step in atherosclerosis is subendothelial retention of LDL-containing lipoproteins [8]. Combined dyslipidemia is highly atherogenic because its subpopulation composition with increased LDL particles and small dense LDL facilitates subendothelial retention by multiple mechanisms. CD is associated with pathologic evidence of atherosclerosis and ultrasound findings of vascular dysfunction in children, adolescents, and young adults. It is also predictive of early clinical cardiovascular events in adult life: in the long-term Princeton Follow-up Study, elevated TG with reduced HDL-C identified at a mean age of 12 years predicted clinical cardiovascular events at late follow-up, three to four decades later [9].

Thus, CD seen with obesity in childhood and adolescence is highly atherogenic, associated with pathologic evidence of vascular dysfunction and atherosclerosis in adolescence and predictive of early clinical CVD events in adult life.

Making the Diagnosis of Combined Dyslipidemia

The most recent NHLBI pediatric guidelines were the first to emphasize the importance of CD as a major risk factor for premature atherosclerotic disease beginning in childhood [1]. The guidelines recommend selective lipid screening when overweight or obesity is first identified: (1) at a BMI at or above the 85th percentile for age/sex; (2) when any other major cardiovascular risk is present; and (3) when there is a family history of early CVD or of treated dyslipidemia. Universal lipid screening is recommended between 9 and 11 years of age and again between 17–21 years of age. While non-fasting measures of total cholesterol, HDL-C and non-HDL-C, are accurate, hypertriglyceridemia can only be accurately identified on a fasting lipid profile (FLP) which is therefore recommended for selective screening in these settings.

- Normative values for the lipid components are shown in Table 7.1. Diagnosis of CD requires an average of a least two fasting TG measurements above the 95th percentile with HDL-C at or below the fifth percentile.
- TG measurement is subject to considerable biologic variability with median variation between measurements of 23.5% compared with only 5–6% for cholesterol and HDL-C, so if the first two TG results are highly disparate, a third fasting measurement is recommended.
- In the typical lipid profile of a youth with CD, TG levels are between 150 and 400 mg/dL and HDL-C is <40 mg/dL. Total cholesterol and LDL-C levels may also be mildly elevated.
- TG levels above 1000 mg/dL are associated with definite risk of acute pancreatitis and require investigation for an underlying genetic trait and specific management to prevent pancreatitis. Rarely, a child with CD will have TG levels above 500 mg/dL and will also be at risk for pancreatitis.
- When the diagnosis of CD is confirmed, specific evaluation for comorbidities is recommended:
- Waist circumference (WC) as a measure of visceral adiposity.
- Assessment of fasting glucose to evaluate glucose intolerance per the recommendations of the American Diabetic Association.
- ALT measurement to check for NAFLD.
- Evaluation for the MetS cluster (i.e., elevated WC, high TG, low HDL, elevated blood pressure, elevated blood sugar).

Tables 7.2 and 7.3 show the screening algorithm for diagnosis of CD from the NHLBI pediatric guidelines Fig. 5.1 and Table 6.2.

There are racial, ethnic, and gender differences in TG levels in childhood and adolescence. African Americans have significantly lower TGs and higher HDL-C levels compared with Hispanics and non-Hispanic whites. With puberty, HDL-C levels drop a mean of 10 mg/dL in males with no change in females, regardless of race/ethnicity [1]. These differences suggest that race-, gender-, and developmental stage-specific cut-points may be needed to optimally identify high TGs and CD but normative tables for American youth based on these factors are not currently available.

Table 7.2 NHLBI evidence-based screening algorithm for combined dyslipidemia in childhood and adolescence

Grades are the results of the evidence review. Recommendations are the consensus of the NHLBI expert panel		
Birth—2 years	No lipid screening	Grade C/recommend
4–6 years	No routine screening	Grade B/recommend
	Selective screening	Grade B/strongly recommend
	→ Fasting lipid profile (FLP) X 2[a], average results if:	
	• Parent, grandparent, aunt/uncle, or sibling with history of premature CV disease[b]	
	• Parent with known dyslipidemia, TC > 240 mg/dL	
	• Child has diabetes, hypertension, obesity (BMI > 95th percentile), or smokes cigarettes	
	• Child has moderate/high-risk medical condition[c]	
9–11 years	Universal screening	Grade B/strongly recommend
	• FLP: LDL-C >130 mg/dL, TG >130 mg/dL, HDL <40 mg/dL → Repeat FLP → Lipid algorithms	
12–16 years	No routine screening[d]	Grade B/strongly recommend
	Selective screening	Grade B/strongly recommend
	→ Measure FLP X 2[e], average results if:	
	• Family history now (+) for CV disease	
	• Parent with dyslipidemia, TC > 240 mg/dL	
	• Patient has diabetes, hypertension, BMI > 95th percentile, cigarette smoker	
	• Patient has moderate/ high-risk medical condition (Table 6.2)	
17–21 years	Universal screening X 1	Grade B/strongly recommend

NHLBI National Heart, Lung, and Blood Institute FLP fasting lipid profile, *CV* cardiovascular, *TC* total cholesterol, *LDL-C* low-density liporotein cholesterol, *TG* triglycerides, *HDL-C* high-density lipoprotein cholesterol, *Non-HDL-C* non-high density lipoprotein cholesterol (TC-HDL-C), *BMI* body mass index

GRADING SYSTEM:

GRADE A: Well-designed randomized controlled trials or diagnostic studies performed on a population similar to the guideline's target population

GRADE B: Randomized controlled trials or diagnostic studies with minor limitations; genetic natural history studies; overwhelmingly consistent evidence from observational studies

GRADE C: Observational studies (case-control and cohort design)

GRADE D: Expert opinion, case reports, reasoning from first principles (bench research or animal studies)

[a]Interval between FLP measurements = after 2 weeks, <3 months; Table 7.1 for interpretation of results; Fig. 8.1 for management

[b]Premature CV disease: Parent, grandparent, aunt/uncle, or sibling with heart attack, angina, stroke, coronary artery graft/stent/angioplasty at <55 years in males <65 years in females

[c]Table 7.3 for moderate/high-risk medical conditions

[d]Routine lipid screening not recommended because LDL-C measurements significantly less sensitive/specific for prediction of adult results during puberty

[e]Table 7.1 for interpretation of results; Fig. 8.1 for management

Table 7.3 Risk conditions for lipid screening

High risk:
• Diabetes mellitus, type 1 and type 2
• Chronic renal disease/end-stage renal disease/postrenal transplant
• Postorthotopic heart transplant
• Kawasaki disease with current aneurysms
Moderate risk:
• Kawasaki disease with regressed coronary aneurysms
• Chronic inflammatory disease (systemic lupus erythematosus, juvenile rheumatoid arthritis)
• Human immunodeficiency virus (HIV) infection
• Nephrotic syndrome

Management of Combined Dyslipidemia

Evidence for Response to Lifestyle Change

A significant body of evidence documents major improvements in CD in response to lifestyle changes including calorie limitation, change in diet composition, and increased activity. In all age groups, even small amounts of weight loss are associated with significant decreases in TGs, often with increases in HDL-C. In adults, weight loss of as little as 5% results in a 20% decrease in TGs and an 8 to 10% increase in HDL-C. In youth, a decrease in BMI z-score of at least 0.15 kg/m2 is associated with significant improvement in triglycerides and HDL-C. As the amount of weight loss increases, the magnitude of TG and HDL-C change increases. On NMR analysis, acute weight loss in children and adolescents has been shown to significantly decrease TGs, small dense LDL-C and LDL particles [2].

Changes in diet composition have also been shown to be effective treatment for high TGs and CD. In light of the strong evidence in children and adults associating excessive sugar intake with obesity and with combined dyslipidemia, decreasing simple carbohydrate intake—especially in the form of added sugars—is an important focus. In adults, a low-carbohydrate diet with monounsaturated fat enrichment significantly decreased TGs by a mean of 63%, with associated increases in HDL-C. One-year follow-up of young children (mean age 21 months) with elevated TGs treated with a diet restricted in sugar and carbohydrates was associated with a significant TG decrease from a mean of 274.1 +/- 13.1 mg/dL before treatment to 88.8 ± 13.3 mg/dL. In adolescents and young adults, low glycemic-load diets are as effective as low-fat diets in achieving weight loss and are associated with decreased TGs and increased HDL-C.

In obese children and adolescents, a low-carbohydrate diet with or without weight loss significantly reduces TGs [10]. These diet composition changes have also been shown to significantly improve the LDL subpopulation pattern. Combined, diet composition changes will lower TGs by at least 20%.

Exercise has also been effective in treating CD in youth, alone and in the context of a weight loss plan. Aerobic activity facilitates the hydrolysis and utilization of triglycerides in skeletal muscle, reducing deposition as adipose tissue. In adults, moderately intense activity vs no activity was associated with 20% lower TGs, with lowest levels in the highest activity subjects. In cross-sectional studies in youth, low cardiorespiratory fitness is a strong predictor of high TGs as part of the MetS cluster, and high fitness is associated with a low metabolic risk score. In randomized controlled trials, aerobic exercise interventions are associated with significant decreases in TG levels and increases in HDL-C, proportionate to training intensity [2].

Several studies have attempted to define the optimal type, volume and intensity of activity required for cardiovascular risk reduction. A systematic review of activity-related benefits concluded that youth aged 5–17 years required at least 60 min of at least moderate intensity activity every day. Aerobic activities should make up the majority, at vigorous intensity whenever possible. These recommendations are very similar to the Physical Activity Guidelines from the U.S. Department of Health and Human Services. Multiple randomized, controlled exercise interventions in obese children have shown benefits in weight management and CD [2].

No studies of youth with high TGs or CD have evaluated clinical cardiovascular events in response to lifestyle changes initiated in childhood. In obese youth with high TGs and CD, diet and exercise intervention studies show that subjects who were successful in weight loss showed improvements in vascular measures. In longitudinal cohort studies, lifestyle interventions have been shown to improve multiple vascular measures and low cardiovascular risk in childhood is significantly predictive of better vascular health in adulthood.

Specific lifestyle and pharmaceutical management plans for CD are described in chap. 8.

Conclusion

In youth, CD is a prevalent, highly atherogenic lipid disorder, almost always associated with obesity. CD is strongly associated with a complex of interrelated risk factors including visceral adiposity, IR/T2DM, NAFLD, and the MetS complex which significantly exponentiate risk for CVD. Presence of CD in childhood is definitively associated with early CV events in adult life.

References

1. Expert Panel on Integrated Guidelines for Cardiovascular Health and Risk Reduction in Children and Adolescents; National Heart, Lung, and Blood Institute. Expert panel on integrated guidelines for cardiovascular health and risk reduction in children and adolescents: summary report. Pediatrics. 2011;128(Suppl 5):S213–56. www.nhlbi.nih.gov/guidelines/cvd_ped/index.htm.
2. Kavey RE. Combined dyslipidemia in children and adolescents. Endotext. South Dartmouth (MA): MD Text.com, Inc.; 2000. www.endotext.org.

3. Shah AS, Wilson DP. Primary hypertriglyceridemia in children and adolescents. J Clin Lipidol. 2015;9(5 Suppl):S20–8. https://doi.org/10.1016/j.jacl.2015.04.004.
4. Ogden CL, Fryar CD, Martin CB, Freedman DS, Carroll MD, Gu Q, Hales CM. Trends in obesity prevalence by race and Hispanic origin—1999–2000 to 2017–2018. JAMA. 2020;324(12):1208–10. https://doi.org/10.1001/jama.2020.14590.
5. Lawrence JM, Divers J, Isom S, et al. Trends in Prevalence of Type 1 and Type 2 Diabetes in Children and Adolescents in the US, 2001-2017. JAMA. 2021;326(8):717–27. https://doi.org/10.1001/jama.2021.11165.
6. Morrison JA, Friedman LA, Gray-McGuire C. Metabolic syndrome in childhood predicts adult cardiovascular disease 25 years later: the Princeton lipid research clinics follow-up study. Pediatrics. 2007;120:340–5.
7. Ikezaki H, Lim E, Cupples LA, Liu CT, Asztalos BF, Schaefer EJ. Small dense low-density lipoprotein cholesterol is the most atherogenic lipoprotein parameter in the prospective Framingham offspring study. J Am Heart Assoc. 2021;10(5):e019140. https://doi.org/10.1161/JAHA.120.019140. Epub 2021 Feb 15.
8. Tabas I, Williams KJ, Boren J. Subendothelial lipoprotein retention as the initiating process in atherosclerosis: update and therapeutic implications. Circulation. 2007;116:1832–44.
9. Morrison JA, Glueck CJ, Horn PS, Yeramaneni S, Wang P. Pediatric triglycerides predict cardiovascular disease events in the fourth to fifth decade of life. Metabolism. 2009;58(9):1277–84.
10. Pratt RE, Kavey RE, Quinzi D. Combined dyslipidemia in obese children: response to a focused lifestyle approach. J Clin Lipidol. 2014;8(2):181–6.

Chapter 8
Approach to Management of Combined Dyslipidemia

Janet Carter and Rae-Ellen W. Kavey

Introduction

This chapter focuses on approaches to management of combined dyslipidemia (CD), the atherogenic pattern of high triglyceride (TG) and reduced high-density lipoprotein cholesterol (HDL-C) described in Chap. 7. CD in youth occurs almost exclusively with obesity, present in 30–60% of obese youth from multiple populations. CD prevalence increases as obesity severity increases. Given this strong association, approaches to healthy lifestyle with weight loss represent a major anchor of CD management [1].

In youth and adults, magnitude of lipid change correlates directly with the amount of weight loss [1]. Changes in diet composition even without weight loss can lower TGs by as much as 20% with change focused on decreasing simple carbohydrate intake, especially added sugars. In young children, a diet restricted in sugar and carbohydrates normalized TGs after 1 year. In obese youth, low carbohydrate/ low glycemic-load diets significantly reduce TGs, with or without weight loss [2]. Exercise is effective in treating CD in youth, alone and in combination with weight loss. Aerobic activity facilitates the hydrolysis and utilization of TGs in skeletal muscle, reducing deposition as adipose tissue. In multiple randomized trials in youth, aerobic exercise interventions significantly decreased TG levels and increased HDL-C, proportionate to training intensity [2].

J. Carter (✉)
Department of Pediatrics, Medical University of South Carolina/Morrison Healthcare, Charleston, SC, USA
e-mail: catjan@musc.edu

R.-E. W. Kavey
Department of Pediatrics, University of Rochester Medical Center, Rochester, NY, USA

A. Ashraf, B. Sunil (eds.), *Pediatric Dyslipidemia*,
https://doi.org/10.1007/978-3-031-24113-0_8

Information regarding medication management is included for the rare situations where lifestyle management has been attempted unsuccessfully or the benefits of beginning a medication outweigh the risks.

Lifestyle Approaches to Obesity and Combined Dyslipidemia

The evidence for lifestyle management of dyslipidemia in adults is strong and has changed little for decades. Less research has been done with children and adolescents, but most lifestyle recommendations for disease prevention and treatment are aimed at families and are thus generalizable. This chapter will serve as a guide for providers to begin the conversation regarding healthy lifestyle habits with patients, but it is advised that a registered dietitian nutritionist be involved early in the process to optimize behavior change [3].

Dietary Components with the Most Significant Impact on Dyslipidemia (Summarized in Table 8.1)

Fats

There was a time when "low fat" was the recommendation for overall wellness, but at least six decades of evidence has helped to clarify the distinct effects of different types of fats on blood lipid levels. **Unsaturated fats:** It is now well known that consumption of polyunsaturated and monounsaturated fats in place of saturated fats or refined carbohydrate sources can have significant beneficial effects on blood lipids [3]. When sources of monounsaturated fats are consumed in place of sources of saturated fat, there is much evidence supporting the likelihood of improved heart disease risk. Sources of monounsaturated fats include many cooking oils (e.g., olive, canola, peanut, sunflower, safflower), avocados, peanut butter, nuts and seeds [3]. Two important polyunsaturated fats are omega 3 and omega 6. These fats are considered "essential", which means that they cannot be created in vivo and must be consumed in the diet. Consuming the recommended amount of omega 3 fats has been shown to increase HLD cholesterol (HDL-C) and lower TGs. Consumption of omega 6 fats may protect against heart disease. Sources of these fats include fatty fish (omega 3) (e.g. salmon, herring, sardines, mackerel) and many cooking oils except saturated fats from plant sources (omega 6) (e.g. safflower, grapeseed, flaxseed, sunflower) [3].

Saturated fats are considered less healthy because consumption of excess amounts can lead to increases in LDL cholesterol (LDL-C). It is generally recommended that saturated fat compose no more than 10% of daily calories (less than 7% in high-risk patients). Specifically, replacing 5% of calories from saturated fat with monounsaturated fats or polyunsaturated fats can lead to a 6.5 g/dL and 9 g/dL decrease in LD-C, respectively [4]. Sources of saturated fat include high-fat animal foods like ground beef and processed meats, cheese, high-fat milk, and ice cream and tropical oils like coconut and palm oils [3].

Table 8.1 Summary of diet recommendations by dietary component [5]

Dietary component	Daily recommendation	Sources	Notes
Unsaturated fat (emphasis on polyunsaturated fats)	20–23% of calories for 2–3-year-olds and 15–25% of calories for 4–18-year-olds	Plant-based cooking oils (except coconut and palm oil), avocado, nuts and nut butters, seeds, fatty fish, plant-based butter alternatives	20–23% of calories is approximately 26–63 g/day, depending on calorie needs
Saturated fat	<10% of calories	High-fat animal foods such as beef, processed meats, cheese and other full-fat dairy products, butter, deep-fried food, coconut oil	10% of calories is approximately 13–27 g/day, depending on calorie needs
Trans fat	None	Sources have largely been eliminated but trace amounts could still be in some processed and prepared foods	Label reading will identify the presence of *trans* fat, including the ingredient label (the presence of partially hydrogenated oils would indicate at least a trace amount of *trans* fat)
Fiber	14 g/1000 calories	Vegetables and fruits (especially those with edible skin or peel), whole grain products, legumes, nuts, seeds	Viscous (soluble) fiber is best for LDL-lowering, but both viscous and non-viscous are helpful in weight management
Added sugar	<10% of calories	Sugar-sweetened beverages, candy and chocolate, pastries, sugar-sweetened cereals, some snack foods	10% of calorie is approximately 30–62 g/day, depending on calorie needs

Trans fats are created during food processing that involves the partial hydrogenation of fat (only trace amounts of *trans* fats are found naturally). There has been indisputable evidence that *trans* fats have drastically detrimental effects on heart health and should be eliminated from the diet altogether. Because of this, legislation has been passed that has essentially eliminated them from the food supply. It is still important for consumers to be diligent when reading food labels and to be sure that there is zero *trans* fat, in addition to looking for "partially-hydrogenated" fats and oils in the ingredient list [3].

Cholesterol

Cholesterol is produced in the liver, but the typical American diet also contains cholesterol. It is yet unclear how much of an impact dietary cholesterol intake has on blood cholesterol, specifically LDL-C, but it is generally recommended to limit intake to no more than 200–300 mg per day. Incidentally, cholesterol is only contained in animal foods, which also tend to be higher in saturated fat, so decreases in saturated fat consumption are usually accompanied by decreases in dietary cholesterol [3].

Fiber

Dietary fiber is the non-digestible portion of food and is a very important component of a healthy eating pattern. Soluble fiber is effective in lowering LDL-C, but both soluble and insoluble fiber consumption can assist in weight management through enhanced satiety, thereby improving CD [3].

Dietary Patterns

While the above information is valuable, it is not necessarily practical in use with families in a clinical setting. Rather than dietary components, recommendations are now focusing on dietary patterns. It is speculated that the synergy of a healthy overall eating pattern like the ones described below outweighs a focus on the individual components (though most of the eating plans favored by clinicians basically adhere to the specifics outlined above regarding the impactful dietary components). The two that are featured in this document are the Mediterranean diet and the DASH diet. These two have been researched extensively and have shown to be the most efficacious of all. Please note that it is not recommended to encourage dieting among children and adolescents, but to emphasize that these are healthy eating patterns and not restrictive diets.

Mediterranean Diet

The Mediterranean diet is characterized by high intake of unsaturated fat, fiber, and plant foods with moderate amounts of fish and poultry and low red and processed meat, dairy, and sweets. There is strong evidence that adherence to this type of eating pattern is not only beneficial in the management of dyslipidemia, but in general health and wellness, with stricter adherence engendering more benefit [6]. Table 8.2 summarizes the key points of the diet, but many sample meal plans can be obtained online.

DASH Eating Pattern

While the DASH eating plan was originally developed to help lower blood pressure, it has been shown to be effective in weight and lipid management, as well. The main characteristics of the DASH eating pattern are high intake of produce, a focus on lean meat, poultry, fish and plant sources of protein, moderate consumption of low-fat/fat-free dairy, and minimal sweets/added sugars. Since its introduction in 1997, numerous studies have supported its health-promoting benefits. The NHLBI Pediatric Guidelines for Cardiovascular Health include a DASH Eating Plan, specially adapted for use in children based on food groups and total energy intake [2]. Table 8.3 provides estimated total energy needs/calorie requirements by activity level for boys and girls from 2 to 18 years of age. This information is used to implement the DASH Eating Plan shown in Table 8.4.

Table 8.2 Summary of key points of Mediterranean diet [6]

Key points	Amounts
Vegetables	≥2 servings per main meal
Fruits	1–2 servings per main meal
Minimally refined breads and cereals	1–2 servings per main meal
Potatoes	≤3 servings per week
Fish/seafood	≥2 servings per week
White meat	2 servings per week
Red meat	<2 servings per week
Processed meat	<2 servings per week
Dairy (preferably low-fat)	2 servings per day
Eggs	2–4 per week
Beans and legumes	≥2 servings per week
Nuts, olives, and seeds	1–2 servings per day
Olive oil	Every main meal
Sweets and added sugar/honey	≤2 servings per week
Of note, wine is also recommended in moderation, but *for adults only*	

Table 8.3 Estimated pediatric calorie requirements (in Kilocalories [kcal]) for gender and age groups at three levels of physical activity[a]. Estimates are rounded to nearest 200 calories and were determined using the Institute of Medicine (IOM) equation

		Activity Level[b, c, d]		
Gender	Age (years)	Sedentary[b]	Moderately Active[c]	Active[d]
Child	2–3	1000	1000–1,400[e]	1000-1400[e]
Female	4-8 9–13 14–18	1200 1600 1800	1400–1600 1600–2000 2000	1400–1800 1800–2200 2400
Male	4–8 9–13 14–18	1400 1800 2200	1400–1600 1800–2200 2400–2800	1600–2000 2000–2600 2800–3200

[a] These levels are based on estimated energy requirements from the IOM dietary reference intakes macronutrients report (2002), calculated by gender, age, and activity level for reference-size individuals. "Reference size," as determined by the IOM, is based on median height and weight for ages up to age 18 years and median height and weight for that height to give a body mass index of 21.5 for adult females and 22.5 for adult males

[b] A sedentary activity level in childhood, as in adults, means a lifestyle that includes only the light physical activity associated with typical day-to-day life

[c] Moderately active in childhood means a lifestyle that includes some physical activity, equivalent to an adult walking about 1.5–3 miles per day at 3–4 miles per hour, in addition to the light physical activity associated with typical day-to-day life

[d] Active means a lifestyle that includes more physical activity, equivalent to an adult walking more than 3 miles per day at 3–4 miles per hour, in addition to the light physical activity associated with typical day-to-day life

[e] The calorie ranges shown recognize the needs of different ages within the group. For growing children and adolescents, more calories are needed at older ages

Table 8.4 DASH eating plan: Servings per day by food group and total energy intake

Food group	1200 calories	1400 calories	1600 calories	1800 calories	2000 calories	2600 calories	Serving sizes	Examples and notes	Significance of Each Food Group to DASH Eating Plan
Grains[a]	4–5	5–6	6	6	6–8	10–11	1 slice bread 1 oz dry cereal[b] ½ cup cooked rice, pasta, or cereal[b]	Whole-wheat bread and rolls, whole-wheat pasta, English muffin, pita bread, bagel, cereals, grits, oatmeal, brown rice, unsalted pretzels and popcorn	Major sources of energy and fiber
Vegetables	3–4	3–4	3–4	4–5	4–5	5–6	1 cup raw leafy vegetable ½ cup cut-up raw or cooked vegetable ½ cup vegetable juice	Broccoli, carrots, collards, green beans, green peas, kale, lima beans, potatoes, spinach, squash, sweet potatoes, tomatoes	Rich sources of potassium, magnesium, and fiber
Fruits	3–4	4	4	4–5	4–5	5–6	1 medium fruit ¼ cup dried fruit ½ cup fresh, frozen, or canned fruit ½ cup fruit juice	Apples, apricots, bananas, dates, grapes, oranges, grapefruit, grapefruit juice, mangoes, melons, peaches, pineapples, raisins, strawberries, tangerines	Important sources of potassium, magnesium, and fiber
Fat-free or low-fat milk and milk products	2–3	2–3	2–3	2–3	2–3	3	1 cup milk or yogurt 1½ oz cheese	Fat-free milk or buttermilk; fat-free, low-fat, or reduced-fat cheese; fat-free/low-fat regular or frozen yogurt	Major sources of calcium and protein
Lean meats, poultry, and fish[c]	3 or less	3–4 or less	3–4 or less	6 or less	6 or less	6 or less	1 oz cooked meats, poultry, or fish 1 egg[d]	Select only lean; trim away visible fats; broil, roast, or poach; remove skin from poultry	Rich sources of protein and magnesium

Nuts, seeds, and legumes	3 per week	3 per week	3–4 per week	4 per week	4–5 per week	1	1/3 cup or 1½ oz nuts 2 Tbsp peanut butter 2 Tbsp or ½ oz seeds ½ cup cooked legumes (dried beans, peas)	Almonds, filberts, mixed nuts, peanuts, walnuts, sunflower seeds, peanut butter, kidney beans, lentils, split peas	Rich sources of energy, magnesium, protein, and fiber
Fats and oils[e]	1	1	2	2–3	2–3	3	1 tsp soft margarine 1 tsp vegetable oil 1 Tbsp mayonnaise 2 Tbsp salad dressing	Soft margarine, vegetable oil (canola, corn, olive, safflower), low-fat mayonnaise, light salad dressing	DASH study had 27% of calories as fat, including fat in or added to foods
Sweets and added sugars	3 or less per week	3 or less per week	3 or less per week	5 or less per week	5 or less per week	≤2	1 Tbsp sugar 1 Tbsp jelly or jam ½ cup sorbet, gelatin dessert 1 cup lemonade	Fruit-flavored gelatin, fruit punch, hard candy, jelly, maple syrup, sorbet and ices, sugar	Sweets should be low in fat

[a] Whole grains are recommended for most grain servings as a good source of fiber and nutrients

[b] Serving sizes vary between ½ cup and 1 1/4 cups, depending on cereal type. Check product's Nutrition Facts label

[c] The Food and Drug Administration (FDA) and the Environmental Protection Agency are advising women of childbearing age who may become pregnant, pregnant women, nursing mothers, and young children to avoid some types of fish and shellfish and eat fish and shellfish that are lower in mercury. For more information, call FDA's food information line toll free at 1–888-SAFEFOOD or visit http://www.cfsan.fda.gov/~dms/admehg3.html

[d] Since eggs are high in cholesterol, limit egg yolk intake to no more than four per week; two egg whites have the same protein content as 1 oz meat

[e] Fat content changes serving amount for fats and oils. For example, 1 Tbsp regular salad dressing = one serving; 1 Tbsp low-fat dressing = one-half serving; 1 Tbsp fat-free dressing = zero servings. Abbreviations: *oz* ounce; *Tbsp* tablespoon; *tsp* teaspoon

Weight Management

While a full discussion of weight management is beyond the scope of this chapter, its impact on CD in children and adolescents cannot be ignored. Healthy, calorie-dense, high-unsaturated-fat foods such as nuts (including peanuts) and avocado have long been considered difficult for those with loss goals to include as part of a calorie-conscious diet. Recent evidence, however, shows consumption of these foods enhances satiety and other post-prandial factors in addition to improving diet quality, especially when consumed in place of carbohydrate sources [7, 8].

Relatively small changes in a child or adolescent's BMI z-score can result in significant improvements in lipid parameters and can be achieved through slightly decreased caloric intake and increased physical activity. A focus on limiting simple carbohydrates and replacing them with complex carbohydrates has been very effective in children with combined dyslipidemia [9]. Table 8.3 outlines age- and gender-specific calorie recommendations for weight maintenance that also take activity level into account. It is important not to encourage "dieting" in children and adolescents, but it is helpful to understand caloric need to build mindfulness and to create a moderate calorie deficit for weight loss.

Special Considerations

Behavior Change

The typical American diet is not much like the Mediterranean nor DASH eating patterns, so helping patients and their families make changes can be challenging. While a comprehensive discussion of behavior change is not within the scope of this guide, a few points may be helpful for beginning the process. It is also important to involve a registered dietitian nutritionist early in the process, as they have specialized training and can spend the necessary time with patients that it takes to realize even small changes in behavior. A clinician in a busy practice could help a patient identify one to two specific, realistic, and measurable goals that they are very confident they can meet at least a few days of the week to start. It is best if all providers can familiarize themselves with the concept and practice of motivational interviewing to help patients to take ownership of their own behavior change. Some families have seemingly insurmountable barriers to change which may include but are not limited to the food environment, time availability and management, mental health, and social support [10]. The best plan for providers is to validate these barriers and other concerns of the patient/family and begin the process of helping them identify solutions, one at a time.

Socioeconomic Concerns

Healthy food is often considered more expensive. Despite a 2012 report from the Economic Research Service of the USDA that found this not to be true, it is important to acknowledge this perception when counseling families about healthier lifestyle habits [11]. This is especially important in weight management since obesity and other health risk profiles disproportionately affect lower income and minority families. A helpful way to address this issue is to validate the family's concerns while suggesting very gradual changes that may save them money. For example, since meat and processed foods are typically the most expensive, encourage families to start by cutting back on both as a first step. Also, the USDA provides healthy meal plans at four different cost levels that can help families get started on healthy habits with less worry about the financial impact.

Management of Combined Dyslipidemia by Activity Enhancement

Aerobic exercise interventions addressing CD reference activity intensity, described as a person's level of effort relative to their own fitness level. On a scale of 0–10, if sitting doing nothing is 0 and the highest possible level is 10, then moderate intensity is a 5 or 6 and is associated with a perceptible increase in heart and breathing rates. Vigorous intensity begins at a level of 7 or 8 and is associated with much faster heart and breathing rates. To achieve activity benefits, youth aged 5–17 years require a minimum of 60 min of at least moderate intensity activity every day with aerobic activity as the majority and vigorous intensity whenever possible [2].

The Physical Activity Guidelines from the U.S. Department of Health and Human Services [12] define recommended activity levels for healthy children by age:

- Preschool-aged children (ages 3–5 years) should be encouraged to move and engage in active play and structured activities (throwing games, bicycle or tricycle riding) throughout the day with a target of 3 h of activity of all intensities.
- Youth aged 6 through 17 years need 60 min per day of moderate and vigorous-intensity physical activity to maintain health. The total amount of activity is more important for achieving health benefits than any specific frequency, intensity, duration, or selection of activities.

With specific reference to improving CD in obese youth, low cardiorespiratory fitness is a consistent strong predictor of high TGs, and high fitness is associated with low TGs. In randomized controlled trials, aerobic exercise interventions significantly decrease TG levels and increase HDL-C, proportionate to training intensity [3]. Using accelerometry, replacement of just 10 min of sedentary time per day with 10 min of moderate-to-vigorous activity is associated with significantly lower TG and insulin levels [13].

No studies of youth with CD have evaluated subsequent cardiovascular events in response to lifestyle changes initiated in childhood. However, in longitudinal cohort studies, low cardiovascular risk in childhood is significantly predictive of better vascular health in adulthood and lifestyle interventions improve vascular measures in children and adults. In obese youth with CD, diet and exercise interventions show improvements in vascular measures in subjects with weight loss. Evidence-based activity recommendations are shown in Table 8.5.

Table 8.5 Evidence-based activity recommendations for management of combined dyslipidemia[a]

Newborn to 12 months	Parents should create an environment that models an active lifestyle with moderate sedentary time	Grade D Recommend
	Supportive actions[b] • No screen time	
1–4 years	Encourage unlimited active playtime in safe, supportive environments	Grade D Recommend
	Limit sedentary time, especially TV/video/phone	Grade D Recommend
	Supportive actions: • Counsel routine activity for parents as role models • Encourage family activity at least once per week • Limit total screen time (TV/video/phone) to 1–2 h/day • For children <2 years, discourage screen time altogether • No TV in child's bedroom	
5–10 years	Moderate-to-vigorous physical activity every day	Grade A Strongly recommend
	Limit daily leisure screen time (TV/video/computer/phone)	Grade B Strongly recommend
	Supportive actions: • Activity/screen time history once per year • Match activity recommendations to energy needs/intake → MD prescription for moderate to vigorous activity,1 h/day, vigorous activity on 3 days/week • Limit media/leisure screen time to 2 h/day • No TV in child's bedroom • Recommend appropriate safety equipment for each sport • Support recommendations for daily physical education in schools	
11–17 years	Moderate-to-vigorous physical activity every day	Grade A Strongly recommend
	Limit leisure screen time (TV/video/computer/phone	Grade B Strongly recommend
	Supportive actions: • Activity/screen time history from adolescent at health supervision visits • Match activity recommendations to energy needs/intake → MD encourage adolescents to aim for 1 h/day of moderate-to-vigorous activity, vigorous activity 3 days/week • Encourage no TV or leisure screen time in bedroom • Limit total leisure screen time to <2 h/day • Encourage involvement in year-round activities • Support continued family activity once a week and/or family support of adolescent's activity choices • Endorse appropriate safety equipment for each sport	

[a] Adapted from the NHLBI Expert Panel Pediatric Guidelines[3]; **grades** reflect the findings of the evidence review; **recommendation levels** are the consensus opinion of the Expert Panel

[b] Supportive actions are consensus suggestions from the Expert Panel, provided to support implementation of the recommendations

Medication Therapy for Combined Dyslipidemia

Pharmacologic therapy is only rarely necessary for the treatment of CD in childhood, so information is limited. If TG levels consistently exceed 1000 mg/dL, usually an indication of an underlying genetic problem, the child is at risk for pancreatitis and consultation with a lipid specialist is recommended. Drugs which could potentially be used for management of CD are described below.

HMG-CoA Reductase Inhibitors (Statins)

In adults with high cholesterol and CD, statin therapy is the standard of care, beneficially lowering low-density lipoprotein cholesterol (LDL-C) and LDL particle levels and improving vascular function and cardiovascular outcomes. In childhood, statin treatment has focused on children with monogenic hypercholesterolemia (FH) in whom statins safely and effectively lower LDL-C and improve LDL-C subpopulation characteristics. A systematic review of statin therapy in more than 1000 children showed no significant statin-related adverse events [2]. Twenty-year follow-up of FH patients who began statin therapy at a mean age of 12 years showed LDL-C levels 32% below baseline with decreased carotid vascular change compared with controls, emphasizing the safety and effectiveness of long-term statin therapy initiated in childhood [14]. Current National Heart, Lung, and Blood Institute guidelines recommend that children with fasting TG levels of 200–499 mg/dL and non-HDL-C > 145 mg/dL, following at least a 6-month trial of lifestyle/diet management, be considered for statin therapy [2]. There are yet no published studies examining statin effects on clinical outcomes in youth with CD, but TG levels typically decrease by 10–15% with statin therapy. A Pediatric Heart Network trial is evaluating lipid and vascular responses to statin therapy in adolescents with obesity and CD; results are anticipated in 2022.

Omega-3 Fish Oil

Omega-3 fish oil therapy has been shown to be safe in adults, but results are variable with a systematic review showing no definitive benefits on serum lipids or cardiovascular disease outcomes. In US adolescents, two randomized, controlled trials of omega-3 fish oil showed no significant decrease in TGs and no change in LDL particle number or size [1]. A recent meta-analysis of 12 trials of fish oil supplementation in obese children and adolescents showed TG levels decreased by a mean of 17 mg/dL, a statistically, but likely not clinically, significant change [15].

A synthetic derivative of the omega-3 fatty acid eicosapentaenoic acid (EPA) has been developed (icosapent ethyl or ethyl eicosapentaenoic acid), marketed as Vascepa. In adults with moderately severe TG elevation, EPA lowered TGs by 33% and was associated with reduced ischemic events [1]. There is no information on use of EPA in youth.

Peroxisome Proliferator-Activated Receptor Agonists (Fibrates)

In adults with CD, fibrates lower plasma TGs by 30–50% and increase HDL-C by 2–20% with improved LDL subclass distribution, decreased LDL particles, and reduced CVD events.

In children, treatment with fibrates in a single randomized trial ($n = 14$) and 3 small case series ($n = 7$, $n = 17$, $n = 47$) showed TG lowering by as much as 54% and 17% increase in HDL-C but with reported side effects. There are no long-term trials of the vascular or clinical response to fibrate treatment in children.

Nicotinic Acid (Niacin)

Niacin (nicotinic acid) effectively lowers total cholesterol, LDL-C, and TG levels and raises HDL-C in adults. In long-term studies from the pre-statin era, nicotinic acid significantly reduced cardiovascular events but recent studies in statin-treated subjects showed no additional benefit with niacin and more serious adverse events [1].

Experience with niacin in children is limited to a single case series which demonstrated a high rate of side effects leading to discontinuation [1]. **Niacin is not currently recommended for treatment of high TGs**.

See Fig. 8.1 Algorithm for overall management of combined dyslipidemia.

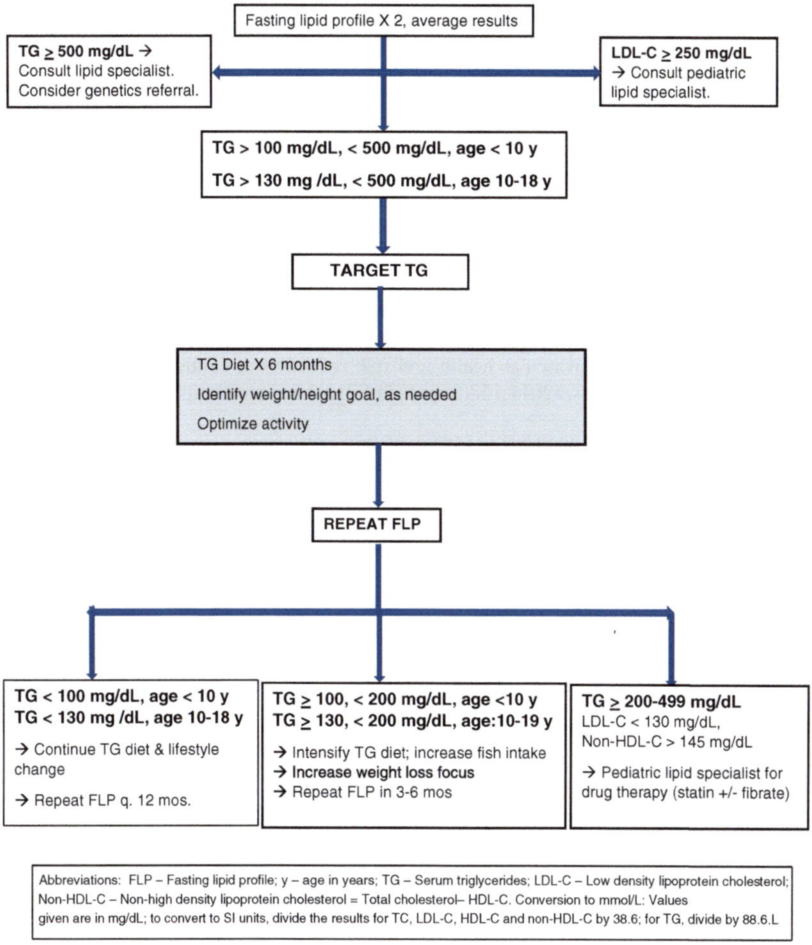

Fig. 8.1 Algorithm for overall management of combined dyslipidemia

Summary

A large body of evidence indicates that a combined diet and activity approach is highly effective for management of CD in youth. The important components of the recommended healthy eating patterns are all very similar: substitute unsaturated fat for saturated fat and refined starches and sugars, increase intake of vegetables and fruits, consume sufficient fiber, and choose lean meats and fat-free dairy when those foods are consumed. Suggested eating patterns and an age-based activity algorithm are provided in this chapter. Evidence for drug therapy of CD in childhood is limited but statins appear to be a logical theoretical choice for the treatment of CD if drug therapy is needed. A decision to initiate drug treatment should only be made in an adolescent with multiple additional high level risk factors after intensive, sustained efforts at lifestyle modification.

References

1. Kavey RE. Combined dyslipidemia in children and adolescents. In: Endotext. South Dartmouth (MA): MD Text.com, Inc.; 2000. www.endotext.org.
2. Expert Panel on Integrated Guidelines for Cardiovascular Health and Risk Reduction in Children and Adolescents; National Heart, Lung, and Blood Institute. Expert panel on integrated guidelines for cardiovascular health and risk reduction in children and adolescents: summary report. Pediatrics. 2011;128(Suppl 5):S213–56. www.nhlbi.nih.gov/guidelines/cvd_ped/index.htm.
3. Eckel RH, Jakicic JM, et al. 2013 AHA/ACC guideline on lifestyle management to reduce cardiovascular risk: a report of the American College of Cardiology/American Heart Association task force on practice guidelines. Circulation. 2014;129(suppl2):S76–S699. https://doi.org/10.1161/01.cir.0000437740.48606.d1.
4. Jacobson TA, Maki KC, et al. National lipid association recommendations for patient-centered management of dyslipidemia: part 2. J Clin Lipidol. 2015;9:S1–S122. https://doi.org/10.1016/j.jacl.2015.09.002.
5. Health and Human Services. Dietary guidelines for Americans, 2020–2025. 9th ed. 2020. DietaryGuidelines.gov. https://www.dietaryguidelines.gov › files › 2020–12.
6. Antoniazzi L, Arroyo-Olivares R, Bittencourt MS, et al. Adherence to a Mediterranean diet, dyslipidemia and inflammation in familial hypercholesterolemia. Nutr Metab Cardiovasc Dis. 2021;31:2014–22.
7. Machado de Souza RG, et al. Nuts and human health outcomes: a systematic review. Nutrients. 2017;9:1311. https://doi.org/10.3390/nu9121311.
8. Park E, et al. Avocado fruit on postprandial markers of cardio-metabolic risk: a randomized controlled dose response trial in overweight and obese men and women. Nutrients. 2018;10:1287. https://doi.org/10.3390/nu10091287.
9. Pratt RE, Kavey RE, Quinzi D. Combined dyslipidemia in obese children: response to a focused lifestyle approach. J Clin Lipidol. 2014;8:181–6. https://doi.org/10.1016/j.jacl.2014.01.003.
10. Cradock KA, Quinlan LR, et al. Identifying barriers and facilitators to diet and physical activity behavior change in type 2 diabetes using a design probe methodology. J Pers Med. 2021;11:72. https://doi.org/10.3390/jpm11020072.
11. Carlson A, Frazão E. Are healthy foods really more expensive? It depends on how you measure the price. U.S. Department of Agriculture, Economic Research Service. 2012: EIB-96.
12. Piercy KL, Troiano RP. Physical activity guidelines for Americans from the US department of health and human services: cardiovascular benefits and recommendations. Circ Cardiovasc Qual Outcomes. 2018;11(11):e005263.
13. Hansen BH, Anderssen SA, Andersen LB, et al. Cross-sectional associations of reallocating time between sedentary and active behaviors on cardiometabolic risk factors in young people: an international children's accelerometry database (ICAD) analysis. Sports Med. 2018;48(10):2401–12. https://doi.org/10.1007/s40279-018-0909-1.
14. Luirink IK, Wiegman A, Kusters DM et al. 20-Year Follow-up of Statins in Children with Familial Hypercholesterolemia. N Engl J Med. 2019;381:1547–56. https://doi.org/10.1056/NEJMoa1816454.
15. Wu S, Zhu C, Wang Z et al. Effects of fish oil supplementation on cardiometabolic risk factors in overweight or obese children and adolescents: a meta-analysis of randomized controlled trials. Front Pediatr. 2021;9:604469. https://doi.org/10.3389/fped.2021.604469.

Chapter 9
Approach to Hypertriglyceridemia

Robert A. Hegele

Case Report

A 3-month-old male of Turkish descent presented for the third time to the emergency department with vomiting, diarrhea, and cough. Previously, pyloric stenosis had been ruled out and a diagnosis of diarrhea with bronchiolitis was made. He was born full term at 37 weeks with Apgar scores of 7 and 9, and a birth weight of 3.37 kg (7.4 lbs., ~50th percentile). There had been no complications during the pregnancy or vaginal delivery. His diet consisted of both breast milk and formula. He was on no medications. On physical examination, he weighed 4.9 kg (10.8 lbs., ~tenth percentile). Fundoscopy revealed no lipemia retinalis. Cardiac and respiratory examinations were unremarkable aside from a mild dry cough. There was mild hepatosplenomegaly without evidence of abdominal pain on palpation. Genitourinary examination was normal. No eruptive xanthomas were seen.

Blood samples were noted by the laboratory to be "creamy" in appearance. Serum lipid profile revealed elevated total cholesterol of 9.85 mmol/L (normal <4 mmol/L), elevated TG of 62.3 mmol/L (normal <1.2 mmol/L), and depressed high-density lipoprotein cholesterol (HDL-C) of 0.55 mmol/L (normal >1 mmol/L). Serum glucose was normal at 5.9 mmol/L. Serum electrolytes, liver enzymes, lipase, and amylase were within normal limits.

The patient was restricted from oral intake and started on intravenous saline. Consequently, serum TG decreased from 62.3 mmol/L at admission to 21.4 mmol/L on day 2 and 12.7 mmol/L on day 3. A low-fat formula containing protein-vitamin-mineral formula component with iron, glucose polymer module, medium-chain TG

R. A. Hegele (✉)
Department of Medicine, Schulich School of Medicine and Dentistry, Western University, London, ON, Canada

Robarts Research Institute, Western University, London, ON, Canada
e-mail: hegele@robarts.ca

A. Ashraf, B. Sunil (eds.), *Pediatric Dyslipidemia*,
https://doi.org/10.1007/978-3-031-24113-0_9

oil, and walnut oil 10 mL/day (essential fatty acids) was gradually introduced by day 7 with further reduction in serum TG to 9.22 mmol/L.

After discharge, he continued on a low-fat diet with medium-chain TG and walnut oil supplementation. There were no further hospital admissions, and specifically, no episodes of pancreatitis. However, due to low nutritional intake, his vertical growth velocity has remained at the tenth percentile with weight velocity below the third percentile. His two healthy brothers aged 6 and 9 years old had normal lipid profiles. His parents were first cousins and were subsequently shown to each have mildly elevated serum TG concentrations. DNA analysis showed the patient was homozygous for the pathogenic rare missense variant p.Gly186Glu in the *LPL* gene-encoding lipoprotein lipase [1].

Hypertriglyceridemia (HTG) in the pediatric population can be stratified into two main clinical entities [2]. First, rare severe HTG is sometimes the result of a monogenic condition called familial chylomicronemia syndrome (FCS), as illustrated by the opening case report. Second, and much more common, is mild-to-moderate HTG in isolation or more often in combination with other lipid disturbances; this condition is multifactorial in nature and is often associated with obesity and insulin resistance [3]. In FCS, the major risk to health is acute pancreatitis, necessitating a distinctive treatment approach both acutely and over the long term. In contrast, for mild-to-moderate HTG, management is geared towards reduction of risk of atherosclerotic cardiovascular disease (ASCVD) later in life. In this chapter, an approach to the child or adolescent with HTG is discussed, with Tables acting as touchpoints along the narrative path. Topics discussed include primary (Tables 9.1 and 9.2) and secondary (Table 9.3) causes of HTG, treatment principles for HTG-associated acute pancreatitis (Table 9.4), general long-term principles of management of HTG (Table 9.5), and current (Table 9.6) and emerging treatments (Table 9.7).

Definition of Hypertriglyceridemia

HTG is commonly encountered, with an abnormal plasma triglyceride (TG) level often as the only finding. Many laboratories report the upper limit of normal for TG as >1.7 mmol/L (>150 mg/dL). Various societies have set different TG intervals to define HTG as either "mild," "moderate," or "severe"; there is no consensus of these levels for adults, much less for children. Severe HTG is often defined as TG >885 mg/dL(>10 mmol/L) or > 1000 mg/dL (>11.1 mmol/L), depending on the favored system of units. Although data for the pediatric population are limited, TG >10 mmol/L may affect in ~1 in 5000 individuals and signals the presence of chylomicrons in serum. TG >2 mmol/L (>175 mg/dL) is seen in 10–15% of children, the clinical consequence being association with deleterious metabolic states such as obesity together with excess risk of future ASCVD. In contrast, for severe TG >10 mmol/L (>885 mg/dL), the main medical concern is increased risk of acute pancreatitis.

Pathophysiology

TG-rich lipoproteins (TRLs)—i.e., chylomicrons and very low-density lipoproteins (VLDL)—are spherical macromolecules comprising core lipids (TG and cholesterol esters) with surface apolipoproteins, phospholipids, and free cholesterol. Exogenous dietary TG circulates in intestine-derived chylomicrons while TG of endogenous origin circulates in liver-derived VLDL. Both chylomicrons and VLDL are cleared by lipoprotein lipase (LPL). Efficiency of both LPL-mediated lipolysis and liver uptake of triglyceride-rich lipoprotein remnants determines fasting and non-fasting TG levels. In mild-to-moderate HTG, increased VLDL production is the commonest initiating factor, while in severe HTG, chylomicron metabolism is disrupted [2].

Several proteins interact with LPL and help regulate its activity [4]. For instance, lipase maturation factor 1 (LMF1) chaperones newly synthesized LPL from the cell interior to the circulation. Glycosylphosphatidylinositol anchored high-density lipoprotein-binding protein 1 (GPIHBP1) anchors LPL to the endothelial surface. Apolipoprotein (apo) C-II and A-V both promote, while apo C-III inhibits LPL activity. The angiopoietin-like proteins, particularly angiopoietin-like protein 3 (ANGPTL3), mainly suppress LPL activity in a tissue-specific manner, and in response to feeding and activity. Mutations in some lipolysis-associated proteins can cause chylomicronemia and are screened for by targeted DNA sequencing panels (see Table 9.1). Some of the lipolysis-associated proteins are molecular targets for new biologic treatments for severe HTG (see Table 9.7).

Children and adolescents with mild-to-moderate HTG often have insulin resistance, obesity, and metabolic syndrome, and sometimes even type 2 diabetes. This milieu drives increased VLDL secretion, due to excessive fatty acids and insulin levels. Insulin resistance and decreased insulin signaling can also lead to increased chylomicron secretion, which can be aggravated by uncontrolled hyperglycemia. Other lipoprotein disturbances in children with HTG include increased non-HDL-C levels since TRL remnants are members of the non-HDL family. Apo B levels are also increased since apo B is a key component of VLDL and TRL remnant particles; apo B levels are a helpful index of atherogenic particle burden. Levels of cholesterol within TRL remnant particles are elevated in HTG; the cholesterol content of remnant particles is much more atherogenic than the TG content. Finally, HDL particles in HTG are qualitatively abnormal and are prone to increased catabolism, leading to reduced HDL-C levels.

Genetics of Hypertriglyceridemia

Primary severe HTG has both monogenic and polygenic determinants [4]. An important example of the former is familial chylomicronemia syndrome (FCS, previously known as hyperlipoproteinemia [HLP] type 1), a rare monogenic condition with estimated prevalence of 1–10 in a million. Diagnosis of this autosomal recessive disorder is based on molecular detection of rare, biallelic (i.e., homozygous or compound heterozygous) variants in one of five genes: *LPL* encoding LPL (accounting for 70–90% of cases), *APOC2*, *APOA5*, *LMF1*, and *GPIHBP1* (Table 9.1). More than 200 different rare pathogenic *LPL* variants have been reported; almost all of these reduce or eliminate LPL activity in the homozygous state, preventing intravascular lipolysis and resulting in accumulation of TG-rich lipoproteins.

Many cases of severe HTG are polygenic in nature, which includes contributions from rare heterozygous variants in the above five FCS genes and/or accumulated common variants at many other loci associated with small increases in TG levels identified in genome-wide association studies (Table 9.1). Also called multifactorial HTG (former hyperlipoproteinemia type 5), secondary factors (Table 9.3) can worsen its severity.

Table 9.1 Primary causes of severe hypertriglyceridemia (TG >10 mmol/L or >885 mg/dL)

1.	Familial chylomicronemia syndrome or monogenic chylomicronemia (formerly HLP type 1 or FCS)
(a)	Lipoprotein lipase (LPL) deficiency due to bi-allelic (two copies) *LPL* gene mutations (70–90% of all cases)
(b)	Glycosylphosphatidylinositol anchored high-density lipoprotein-binding protein 1 (GPIHBP1) deficiency due to bi-allelic *GPIHBP1* gene mutations (5% of cases)
(c)	Apo A-V deficiency due to bi-allelic *APOA5* gene mutations (2–5% of cases)
(d)	Apolipoprotein (apo) C-II deficiency due to bi-allelic *APOC2* gene mutations (2% of cases)
(e)	Lipase maturation factor 1 (LMF1) deficiency due to bi-allelic *LMF1* gene mutations (1–2% of cases)
2.	Multifactorial or polygenic chylomicronemia (formerly HLP type 5 or mixed hyperlipidemia)
(a)	Complex genetic susceptibility, including: • Heterozygous (i.e., single copy) rare large-effect gene variants for monogenic chylomicronemia (see above 5 genes) seen in 15–20% of cases • Accumulated common small-effect TG-raising polymorphisms (e.g., numerous GWAS loci including *APOA1-C3-A4-A5*; *TRIB1*, *LPL*, *MLXIPL*, *GCKR*, *FADS1–2-3*, *NCAN*, *APOB*, *PLTP*, *ANGPTL3*)
3.	Other rare genetic conditions
(a)	Transient infantile HTG (glycerol-3-phosphate dehydrogenase 1 deficiency) due to bi-allelic *GPD1* gene mutations (<5 families so far reported)

Mild-to-moderate HTG is also polygenic in nature (Table 9.2). At the genomic level, isolated HTG (former type HLP 4) resembles severe HTG but has a lower total burden of genetic determinants. Dysbetalipoproteinemia (former type HLP 3) also has a polygenic foundation but has in addition homozygosity for the binding defective apo E2/E2 isoform or a rare binding-defective dominant mutation in the *APOE* gene. Combined hyperlipidemia (former HLP type 2B) is another polygenic trait that resembles isolated HTG at the DNA level. Secondary factors (Table 9.3) are important contributors to clinical expression to all forms of HTG that have a polygenic basis.

Table 9.2 Primary causes of mild-to-moderate HTG (TG 2.0–9.9 mmol/L or 175–885 mg/dL)

1. Multifactorial or polygenic HTG (formerly HLP type 4 or familial HTG)
(a) Complex genetic susceptibility, including:
• Heterozygous (i.e., single copy) rare large-effect gene variants for monogenic chylomicronemia (see above 5 genes) seen in 15–20% of cases; and/or
• Accumulated common small-effect TG-raising polymorphisms (e.g. numerous GWAS loci including *APOA1-C3-A4-A5*; *TRIB1*, *LPL*, *MLXIPL*, *GCKR*, *FADS1–2-3*, *NCAN*, *APOB*, *PLTP*, *ANGPTL3*)
2. Dysbetalipoproteinemia (formerly HLP type 3 or dysbetalipoproteinemia)
(b) Complex genetic susceptibility (see above) plus
• *APOE* E2/E2 homozygosity
• *APOE* dominant rare variant heterozygosity
3. Combined hyperlipoproteinemia (formerly HLP type 2B or familial combined hyperlipidemia)
Complex genetic susceptibility (see above)

Secondary Causes of Hypertriglyceridemia

In children as in adults, secondary factors are important contributors in many cases of HTG. Some of these are shown in Table 9.3. As in adults, obesity from a poor diet and inactivity is common, as already mentioned, and will be discussed in greater depth below. In the assessment of a child or adolescent with severe dyslipidemia, it is important to exclude additional secondary causes, such as type 2 diabetes, hypothyroidism, liver or renal disease, autoimmune disorders, and certain medications associated with lipid perturbations [5]. Some secondary causes can themselves result from genetic predisposition, for example, abdominal obesity, metabolic syndrome, and type 2 diabetes. However, routine genetic testing is currently not recommended for any of these secondary causes.

Table 9.3 Secondary causes of hypertriglyceridemia

Diet with high-positive energy-intake balance and high fat or high glycemic index
Increased alcohol consumption (>1 and >2 units daily, respectively, for women and men)
Obesity, especially central or visceral obesity
Metabolic syndrome
Insulin resistance
Diabetes mellitus (predominantly type 2)
Hypothyroidism
Renal disease (proteinuria, uremia, or glomerulonephritis)
Pregnancy (particularly in the third trimester)
Paraproteinemia, myeloma
Systemic lupus erythematosus
Sarcoidosis
HIV infection
Medications: • Glucocorticoids • Oral estrogen • Tamoxifen • Thiazide diuretics • Non-cardioselective beta-blockers • 13-cis-retinoic acid (Accutane) • Bexarotene • Propofol • Bile acid sequestrants • Cyclophosphamide • L-asparaginase • Capecitabine • Interferons • Protease inhibitors • Atypical antipsychotic agents (such as clozapine and olanzapine)

Severe Monogenic Hypertriglyceridemia: Familial Chylomicronemia Syndrome

Fasting plasma TG levels >10 mmol/L (>885 mg/dL) in children can indicate the pathological presence of chylomicrons. Chylomicronemia in pediatric patients is typically a monogenic autosomal recessive disorder that is most often due to inherited deficiency of either LPL or one of the activating proteins or binding partners discussed above. Collectively, these conditions are referred to as FCS. Levels of other lipoproteins, such as low-density lipoprotein (LDL) and HDL are often low because of impaired intravascular processing of TRLs to smaller lipoproteins.

Clinical features of chylomicronemia include failure to thrive in infants, eruptive xanthomas, lipemia retinalis, hepatosplenomegaly, recurrent abdominal pain, nausea and vomiting, and risk of acute pancreatitis. Less common clinical features include intestinal bleeding, pallor, anemia, irritability, diarrhea, seizures, and encephalopathy. Eruptive xanthomas are raised clusters of small yellowish-orange papules that appear on the torso, back, buttocks, shoulders, and thighs. They may arise suddenly and then recede over weeks as TG levels fall. Lipemia retinalis refers to retinal vessels that appear white or pink on fundoscopic examination, occurring with TG >33 mmol/L (>3000 mg/dL). Vision is unaffected. Hepatosplenomegaly is also related to the degree of TG elevation and is reversible as levels improve.

Risk of acute pancreatitis increases markedly with TG >10 mmol/L (>885 mg/dL), rising sharply with TG >20 mmol/L (>1770 mg/dL). Pancreatitis due to HTG is sometimes fatal. Complications include chronic pancreatitis, pancreatic insufficiency, pancreatic necrosis, pancreatic abscess, or pancreatic pseudocyst. Pancreatitis is hypothesized to result from pathological release of exocrine lipase into local capillaries, resulting in aberrant lipolysis and generation of toxic inflammatory lipid species, which in turn promote autodigestion of the pancreas. A clinical rule of thumb is that pancreatitis risk is markedly reduced after achieving TG levels <500 mg/dL (<5.6 mmol/L).

Traditional biochemical assays for LPL deficiency have not always been reliable or reproducible. Direct gene sequencing is the preferred diagnostic method to detect bi-allelic mutations in the five canonical genes for FCS—i.e., *LPL*, *APOC2*, *APOA5*, *LMF1*, and *GPIHBP1*. Genetic testing for FCS is becoming more accessible and should be performed if the diagnosis of FCS is suspected.

Other Monogenic Disorders Associated with Hypertriglyceridemia

Inherited lipodystrophies can indirectly result in severe HTG. These rare monogenic conditions present with a range of clinical features, including loss and redistribution of adipose tissue plus insulin resistance leading to severe diabetes. Young patients with severe lipodystrophy presentations can have chylomicronemia and acute pancreatitis. Also, children with hepatic glycogen storage disease have HTG through a distinct enzymatic mechanism (glucose-6-phosphatase deficiency); treatment requires continuous complex carbohydrate feeding regimens prescribed as frequent meals usually delivered by enteral feeding tube and supplementation with corn-starch overnight.

Polygenic or Multifactorial Chylomicronemia

In contrast to rare monogenic syndromes, many patients with severe HTG do not have a single genetic determinant but instead have polygenic or multifactorial chylomicronemia syndrome (MCS; formerly HLP type 5). In MCS, patients have an excess of small-effect common TG-raising genetic variants that either increase production or decrease catabolism of circulating TRLs, or both. An individual's total burden of these numerous small effect genetic variants can be quantified using a polygenic score.

In adults with TG >885 mg/dL (10 mmol/L), targeted DNA sequencing indicates that high polygenic risk is at least 50- to 100-times more common than FCS due to bi-allelic rare mutations. Although children have not been studied systematically, many cases of pediatric severe HTG may likewise similarly result from a high burden of polygenic variants rather than from FCS. Polygenic scores for dyslipidemia are currently a research tool and are not ready for clinical use although they may one day prove to be useful. In adults with MCS, a secondary non-genetic factor frequently forces expression of the genetic susceptibility. This is likely to also be the case in children, with obesity being an example.

Combined Hyperlipidemia

Combined hyperlipidemia (CHL, formerly HLP type 2B) is characterized by concurrently elevated total and LDL cholesterol and TG all >90th percentile for age and sex in probands and relatives. Elevated TG is due to VLDL and not chylomicrons. ASCVD risk in CHL is related to the degree of LDL-C and TG elevation, which is integrated by the number of apo B-containing particles. Indeed, non HDL-C and apo B levels are superior to LDL-C in predicting ASCVD risk; both are more accurate laboratory measures than LDL-C and do not require fasting, making them more practical in the clinical setting.

Like MCM, CHL is a complex trait that results from accumulation of numerous small-effect common alleles from many different chromosomes and genetic loci encoding a range of gene products that raise TG and LDL-C levels. There are also important contributions from secondary factors. There are no published guidelines or best practice statements for management of children with the CHL profile. Because elevated LDL-C is a core biochemical feature, statin treatment may be a consideration, especially with a positive family history of premature ASCVD. Treatment of HTG would center on non-pharmacologic approaches.

Obesity-Associated Dyslipidemia

Children are increasingly presenting with obesity-associated dyslipidemia, which includes HTG, elevated small dense LDL particles, depressed HDL-C levels, and increased apo B. Obesity-associated dyslipidemia overlaps phenotypically with CHL, is associated with increased risk of ASCVD and is considered to be a target for treatment [5]. In the absence of modifiable secondary causes of HTG, lifestyle, or non-pharmacologic management is the cornerstone (Table 9.5).

Approach to the Patient with HTG-Associated Pancreatitis (Table 9.4)

Table 9.4 Treatment for hypertriglyceridemia-associated acute pancreatitis

Intervention	Rationale	Comment
NPO; cessation of oral intake for several days	To interrupt the supply of substrate used to generate chylomicrons, thus allowing for residual lipolytic and non-lipolytic capacity to hydrolyze and clear large TG-rich particles	Currently, the most effective acute intervention, with 50% reduction in plasma TG levels within 24–36 h, which is predictable and reliable based on lipoprotein metabolism and physiology
IV hydration with saline or Ringer's lactate	Pancreatitis is often associated with volume depletion, which is further exacerbated by being NPO; hydration using non-glucose containing repletion fluids is preferred	Glucose alone in IV repletion fluid may be used by the liver in the de novo production of endogenous TG-rich lipoproteins
Pain management	May be transiently required in the context of acute pancreatitis	To be used with circumspection and clinical judgment
Insulin	Only if there is accompanying hyperglycemia or uncontrolled diabetes	Use of insulin in normoglycemic individuals presents risk of hypoglycemia; there is minimal evidence that insulin in this situation improves long-term outcomes
Apheresis	To physically extract large TG-rich lipoproteins and potentially toxic fatty acids and pro-inflammatory molecules	Invasive, costly treatment that is not risk free and offers no evidence-based benefit over NPO and hydration in this situation

TG triglyceride, *IV* intravenous, *NPO* nil per os (nothing by mouth)

HTG underlies up to 15% of pancreatitis cases. Initial diagnostic and therapeutic steps should be the same as in other causes of pancreatitis. A TG level should be determined in all children with acute pancreatitis; severe HTG may be present even when the primary cause seems obvious. Initially, intravenous (IV) glucose should be avoided as this may further increase TG levels. HTG-associated pancreatitis should generally be managed supportively and conservatively, by withholding oral intake and administration of IV fluids. TG levels rapidly fall following cessation of oral intake, with a half-life of ~30 h. Insulin infusions, heparin or apheresis have also been proposed to rapidly lower TG, but there is no definitive evidence that these measures are superior to conservative management.

General Non-pharmacologic Approaches to HTG (Table 9.5)

Table 9.5 General principles for management of mild-to-moderate hypertriglyceridemia

Intervention	Details	Comment
Meal scheduling and hygiene	Eat breakfast daily; establish a steady schedule of meals; limit meals outside the home; eat in the kitchen/dining room, never in front of television or computer; family meals at least five times a week	Positive behavioral changes around meals and diet to ensure lifelong constructive attitude towards nutrition that remains the foundation of care
Dietary fat modification	25–30% of calories from fat; ≤7% from saturated fat; ~10% from monounsaturated fat; <200 mg/day of cholesterol; avoid trans fat	Reduces substrate for synthesis of TG-rich lipoproteins
Carbohydrate modification	Promote complex carbohydrates; limit simple carbohydrates	Improved glycemic index; reduces TG-rich lipoprotein production; reduces insulin resistance
Beverages	Avoid sweetened beverages; water is best for children	Improved glycemic index; reduces TG-rich lipoprotein production; reduces insulin resistance
Fruits and vegetables	Consume ≥5 servings of fruits and vegetables a day	Improved glycemic index; reduces TG-rich lipoprotein production; reduces insulin resistance
Physical activity	1 h of moderate-vigorous physical activity 6 days per week; promote walking or cycling to school; activities should involve parents or friends; promote even small amounts of moderate to vigorous activities; promote enjoyable and fun activities	Activity improves lipolysis and fatty acid utilization, reduces insulin resistance and is important in weight maintenance
Sedentary behavior	Limit screen time ≤ 2 h per day Restrict access to gaming and internet after bedtime	As part of rebalancing of activity versus inactivity
Parental and family involvement	Allow children to self-regulate meals; avoid overly restrictive behaviors; parents engaged in grocery shopping and meal preparation; counsel patient and family for healthy eating behaviors; parents serve as a role model; parents should encourage their child and give positive feedback; lifestyle tips are aimed at the entire household	Support from parents and family is important in reinforcing and maintaining positive diet, activity, and lifestyle changes
Alcohol	Should be strictly avoided	Inhibits lipolysis, increase production of hepatic TG-rich lipoproteins

Epidemiological studies show that patients with mild-to-moderate HTG are at increased risk of ASCVD. In patients with mild-to-moderate HTG, it is therefore reasonable to reduce both atherogenic VLDL and associated risk factors by non-pharmacologic means where possible. This can best be achieved by identification and treatment of any underlying cause of elevated TG (see Table 9.3). The same initial approach applies to patients with severe HTG as most of these patients also have multiple risk factors and are at risk of developing ASCVD.

It is reasonable to start with non-pharmacologic treatment where possible (see Table 9.3). Non-pharmacologic management in all HTG patients includes: (1) avoidance of simple carbohydrates; (2) low-fat diet (<30% of total daily caloric intake) and when TG level > 885 mg/dL (10 mmol/L), a very low-fat diet (<15% of total daily caloric intake); (3) weight loss in patients who are overweight or obese; (4) strict glycemic control in patients with diabetes or impaired glucose metabolism; (5) limitation or abstinence of alcohol if appropriate; and (6) addressing any other secondary causes (Table 9.3).

Individuals with FCS are a special case because of the genetic deficiency of lipolytic capacity that makes patients more resistant to non-pharmacologic approaches [6]. FCS patients must follow a stringent low-fat diet (e.g., <15% of daily caloric intake from fat), which presents a challenge over a lifetime. Medium-chain fatty acids can provide an alternate source of dietary fat given their direct absorption into the portal circulation with no reliance on chylomicron formation. Supplementation with essential fatty acids (such as walnut oil or sunflower oil topically) can be considered.

Drug Treatment for Severe HTG (Table 9.6)

To prevent acute pancreatitis, some guidelines suggest reducing TG to <500 mg/dL (<5.6 mmol/L) [7]. This reduction can be partially achieved by the above non-pharmacologic approaches, implementing a very low-fat diet, and then by adding fibrates and/or omega-3 fatty acids for patients with persistently severe HTG [8]. In cases of obesity-associated severe HTG after failure of lifestyle measures, a trial of a TG-lowering agent such as icosapent ethyl or fibrate could be considered, beginning with the lowest available dose (e.g., fenofibrate 100 mg daily) while monitoring for adverse effects.

Table 9.6 Established treatments for hypertriglyceridemia

Treatment	Rationale	Comment
Fibrates	Agonists of PPAR-alpha with multiple TG-lowering effects on both production and catabolism	Minimally effective to ineffective in FCS; they can lower TG by 50% in other forms of HTG; their role in ASCVD prevention remains to be determined
Omega-3 fatty acids	Poorly defined mechanism of TG lowering, but these are considered relatively safe	Minimally effective to ineffective in FCS; they can lower TG by 20–30% in other forms of HTG; over the counter forms have questionable value; icosapent ethyl has been shown to prevent ASCVD when added to statin
Statins	Inhibitors of HMG-CoA reductase that primarily reduce LDL-C	Secondarily can reduce TG by 10–15% but are minimally effective in and not indicated for severe HTG
Ezetimibe	Blocks intestinal sterol absorption via NPC1L1 that primarily reduces LDL-C	Secondarily can reduce TG by 5–10% but are minimally effective in and not indicated for severe HTG
PCSK9 inhibitors	Inhibitors of proprotein convertase subtilisin kexin type 9 that primarily reduce LDL-C	Secondarily can reduce TG by 10–15% but are minimally effective in and not indicated for severe HTG
Niacin	Pleiotropic effect on lipid profile	Can reduce TG by up to 40% but use has declined due to adverse effects and neutral impact on clinical outcomes

ASCVD atherosclerotic cardiovascular disease, *FCS* familial chylomicronemia syndrome, *HMG-CoA* 3-hydroxymethyl-glutaryl-coenzyme A, *HTG* hypertriglyceridemia, *LDL-C* low-density lipoprotein cholesterol, *NPC1L1* Niemann-Pick C1 like protein 1, *PCSK9* proprotein convertase subtilisin kexin-9, *PPAR* peroxisomal proliferator-activated receptor, *TG* triglyceride

Fibric Acid Derivatives (Fibrates)

Fibric acid derivatives or fibrates, such as gemfibrozil, fenofibrate, or bezafibrate, can reduce plasma TG by 50–70%, and can raise plasma HDL-C by up to 20% [8]. These are currently the most reliable pharmacological therapies to reduce TG. If a fibrate is necessary in a patient already being treated with a statin, fenofibrate, and bezafibrate are safer to use than gemfibrozil, with lower risk of statin associated muscle complications. Fibrates modulate activity of hepatic peroxisome proliferator-activated receptor (PPAR)-alpha, increasing fatty acid oxidation and reducing VLDL production.

Fibrates approved for use in adults have limited clinical trial evidence in children. Few adult trials have shown benefit of fibrates on ASCVD event reduction; the primary indication would be prophylaxis of pancreatitis. Fibrates are thus mainly reserved for the treatment of patients with severe HTG to reduce risk of acute pancreatitis and can also be considered as add-on therapy for patients with high ASCVD risk who may need a second agent because TG remains markedly elevated. There is no regulator-based indication for such treatment in patients <18 years; more research is desirable to generate higher quality evidence through appropriate clinical trials in children and adolescents. An ongoing randomized

ASCVD outcome trial of pemafibrate—a novel selective peroxisome proliferator-activated receptor modulator—has enrolled adult statin-treated patients with type 2 diabetes and TG between 2.3 and 5.4 mmol/L (200 and 475 mg/dL), was terminated due to lack of efficacy.

Omega-3 Fatty Acids

In 2018, the multinational REDUCE-IT trial of icosapent ethyl, which is purified eicosapentanoic acid, showed a 25% relative risk reduction in primary ASCVD end point, corresponding to a number needed to treat of 21 patients to prevent one event. However, a subsequent study that used a mixture of omega-3 fatty acids was negative with respect to ASCVD outcomes, suggesting that purified icosapent ethyl might have unique and pleiotropic effects to reduce ASCVD risk. Current treatment guidelines in adults now advise that for statin treated patients with residual HTG up to 5.6 mmol/L (500 mg/dL), icosapent ethyl 4 g daily can be added to reduce ASCVD risk; a similar strategy could be considered in older children with HTG. In contrast, other omega-3 preparations, including over the counter supplements are explicitly discouraged in this context.

Other Available Therapies (Table 9.6)

Statins are primarily low-density lipoprotein (LDL)-lowering drugs that only modestly (5–15%) lower TG; however, statins are central to ASCVD risk reduction. Niacin, ezetimibe, and PCSK9 inhibitor therapy are not recommended for patients with severe HTG. Bile acid sequestrants should be avoided in children with HTG due to their potential to further increase TG levels. Plasmapheresis or plasma exchange are generally not recommended for patients with severe HTG, even during episodes of acute pancreatitis. Worth mentioning in the context of severe HTG is lomitapide, which is a microsomal triglyceride transfer protein inhibitor that is currently approved for the treatment of adult homozygous familial hypercholesterolemia (HoFH). However, anecdotal evidence suggests that lomitapide may be useful in treating FCS that is refractory to traditional therapies although further study is required.

Targeting Apolipoprotein C-III: Volanesorsen; olezarsen; AROAPOC3 (Table 9.7)

Apolipoprotein (apo) C-III is a 79 amino acid protein with pleiotropic effects in lipoprotein metabolism that is a well-validated treatment target for both severe and mild-to-moderate HTG to prevent acute pancreatitis and ASCVD, respectively [9]. The antisense oligonucleotide (ASO) RNA drug volanesorsen (Waylivra, Akcea

Table 9.7 Emerging treatments for hypertriglyceridemia

Name	Mechanism of action	Possible indication	Stage	Biochemical effect
Pemafibrate	Selective PPAR modulator	Elevated TG; no reduction in ASCVD	Phase 3; program terminated	Reduces TG, increases HDL-C
Volanesorsen (Waylivra)	First-generation anti-APOC3 ASO	FCS	Approved in Europe but not North America	Reduces TG, increases HDL-C
Olezarsen or AKCEA-APOCIII-L_{Rx}	GalNac-conjugated anti-APOC3 ASO	FCS; severe HTG; ASCVD	Phase 3	Reduces TG, increases HDL-C
ARO-APOC3	Short interfering RNA	FCS; severe HTG; ASCVD	Phase 2–3	Reduces TG, increases HDL-C
Evinacumab	Anti-ANGPTL3 antibody	FH; severe HTG; FCS; homozygous FH	Phase 3	Reduces TG, LDL-C, and HDL-C
Vupanorsen or IONIS-ANGPTL3-L_{Rx}	GalNac-conjugated anti-ANGPTL3 ASO	FH; severe HTG; FCS; homozygous FH	Phase 3; program terminated	Reduces TG, LDL-C, and HDL-C
ARO-ANG3	Short interfering RNA	FH; severe HTG; FCS; homozygous FH	Phase 2–3	Reduces TG, LDL-C, and HDL-C

APOC3 apolipoprotein C-III, *ASCVD* atherosclerotic cardiovascular disease, *ANGPTL3* angiopoietin like 3, *ASO* antisense oligonucleotide, *FCS* familial chylomicronemia syndrome, *FH* familial hypercholesterolemia, *GalNac* N-acetylgalactosamine, *HDL-C* high-density lipoprotein cholesterol, *HoFH* homozygous FH, *HTG* hypertriglyceridemia, *LDL-C* low-density lipoprotein cholesterol, *PPAR* peroxisome proliferator-activated receptor

Pharmaceuticals) reduces apo C-III. In the APPROACH study (A Study of ISIS 304801 in Patients With Familial Chylomicronemia Syndrome) and the COMPASS study (A Study of Volanesorsen in Patients With Hypertriglyceridemia), at 3 months, patients on volanesorsen had −77% and −71% decreases in plasma TG levels, respectively, plus favorable changes across the lipid profile. However, in FCS patients, volanesorsen was associated with thrombocytopenia. In August 2018, the US Food and Drug Administration (FDA) failed to approve volanesorsen. In contrast, the European Medicines Agency has approved volanesorsen for FCS with some caveats. Development of a next-generation N-acetylgalactosamine (GalNac)-conjugated ASO targeting apo C-III, namely olezarsen (formerly AKCEA-APOCIII-LRx), appears to mitigate thrombocytopenia risk while preserving beneficial effects. Also, a promising siRNA molecule called AROAPOC3 (Arrowhead Pharmaceuticals) that is currently in early phase clinical trials seems to avoid this risk while retaining the metabolic benefits of targeting apo C-III.

Targeting Angiopoietin-Like Protein 3: Evinacumab, vupanorsen, and AROANG3 (Table 9.7)

ANGPTL3 is a liver-derived protein that broadly regulates lipid metabolism, primarily through inhibiting plasma lipases. Evinacumab, a monoclonal antibody that targets ANGPTL3 [9] was approved in February 2021 by the US FDA an adjunct to other LDL-C lowering therapies for adult and pediatric patients >12 years with HoFH and also received a positive opinion in 2021 from the European Medicines Agency. Interestingly, preliminary data indicate that evinacumab is minimally effective in FCS, although it does lower triglycerides in adults with severe HTG that is not due to FCS.

Vupanorsen is a GalNac-modified ASO targeting ANGPTL3, which in a dose-ranging study in patients with mild HTG and fatty liver showed reductions in plasma TG and LDL cholesterol of 44% and 7%, respectively, although development was halted due to concerns over hepatotoxicty. Early efficacy studies of the short interfering RNA AROANG3 (Arrowhead Pharmaceuticals) apparently show similar efficacy across the lipoprotein profile with no safety issues so far.

Summary

HTG in the pediatric population presents unique challenges compared to adults. FCS is genetic, predisposes to the serious complication of acute pancreatitis and is refractory to non-pharmacologic and existing pharmacologic therapies. Fortunately, new treatment options, particularly inhibitors of apo C-III may offer enhanced levels of efficacy and safety that give hope to FCS patients. In more common mild-to-moderate multifactorial HTG, genetic factors also play a role, but secondary factors, particularly obesity, are important determinants in the children and adolescents. The risk to these patients is ASCVD rather than pancreatitis. Overall, multifactorial HTG patients respond better than FCS patients to non-pharmacologic interventions and existing treatments, but emerging therapies might prove to be helpful in many patients with HTG regardless of etiology.

Acknowledgments None.

Financial Support and Sponsorship: R.A.H. is supported by the Jacob J. Wolfe Distinguished Medical Research Chair, the Edith Schulich Vinet Canada Research Chair in Human Genetics, the Martha G. Blackburn Chair in Cardiovascular Research and operating grants from the Canadian Institutes of Health Research (Foundation Grant) and the Heart and Stroke Foundation of Ontario (G-21-0031455) and the Academic Medical Association of Southwestern Ontario (INN21–011).

Conflicts of Interest R.A.H. reports consulting fees from Acasti, Akcea/Ionis, Amgen, Arrowhead, Boston Heart, HLS Therapeutics, Novartis, Pfizer, Regeneron, Sanofi and UltraGenyx.

References

1. Rahalkar AR, Giffen F, Har B, Ho J, Morrison KM, Hill J, Wang J, Hegele RA, Joy T. Novel LPL mutations associated with lipoprotein lipase deficiency: two case reports and a literature review. Can J Physiol Pharmacol. 2009;87:151–60.
2. Berberich AJ, Hegele RA. A modern approach to dyslipidemia. Endocr Rev. 2021;43:611. https://doi.org/10.1210/endrev/bnab037.
3. Lazarte J, Hegele RA. Pediatric dyslipidemia-beyond familial hypercholesterolemia. Can J Cardiol. 2020;36:1362–71.
4. Dron JS, Hegele RA. Genetics of hypertriglyceridemia. Front Endocrinol. 2020;11:455.
5. Ashraf AP, Sunil B, Bamba V, Breidbart E, Brar PC, Chung S, Gupta A, Khokhar A, Kumar S, Lightbourne M, Kamboj MK, Miller RS, Patni N, Raman V, Shah AS, Wilson DP, Kohn B. Case studies in pediatric lipid disorders and their management. J Clin Endocrinol Metab. 2021;106(12):3605–20. https://doi.org/10.1210/clinem/dgab568.
6. Williams L, Rhodes KS, Karmally W, Welstead LA, Alexander L, Sutton L. Familial chylomicronemia syndrome: bringing to life dietary recommendations throughout the life span. J Clin Lipidol. 2018;12:908–19.
7. Grundy SM, Stone NJ, Bailey AL, Beam C, Birtcher KK, Blumenthal RS, Braun LT, de Ferranti S, Faiella-Tommasino J, Forman DE, Goldberg R, Heidenreich PA, Hlatky MA, Jones DW, Lloyd-Jones D, Lopez-Pajares N, Ndumele CE, Orringer CE, Peralta CA, Saseen JJ, Smith SC Jr, Sperling L, Virani SS, Yeboah J. 2018 AHA/ACC/AACVPR/AAPA/ABC/ACPM/ADA/AGS/APhA/ASPC/NLA/PCNA guideline on the Management of Blood Cholesterol: a report of the American College of Cardiology/American Heart Association task force on clinical practice guidelines. Circulation. 2019;139:e1082–143.
8. Laufs U, Parhofer KG, Ginsberg HN, Hegele RA. Clinical review on triglycerides. Eur Heart J. 2020;41:99–109c.
9. D'Erasmo L, Bini S, Arca M. Rare treatments for rare dyslipidemias: new perspectives in the treatment of homozygous familial hypercholesterolemia (HoFH) and familial chylomicronemia syndrome (FCS). Curr Atheroscler Rep. 2021;23:65.

Chapter 10
Lipoprotein (a) [Lp(a)]

Mostafa Salama and Seema Kumar

Case Scenarios

Question 1. A 12-year-old boy was recently adopted with an unknown family history. His body mass index (BMI) is at the 87th percentile and his blood pressure is normal. A low-density lipoprotein cholesterol (LDL-C) is 70 mg/dL. Lipoprotein(a) level is 500 nmol/L. Of the following, the most accurate statement regarding his risk for atherosclerotic cardiovascular disease (ASCVD) is:

A. At risk category since LDL cholesterol is normal
B. High risk since lipoprotein(a) is extremely high
C. Intermediate risk as BMI is in the overweight category
D. Low risk since blood pressure and LDL cholesterol are normal

Answer: A

Critique: Patients with elevated lipoprotein(a) levels (> 50 mg/dL or > 125 nmol/L) are at increased risk for atherosclerotic cardiovascular disease (ASCVD) events including myocardial infarction, ischemic stroke, valvular aortic stenosis, and cardiovascular mortality. The boy in the vignette has an extremely elevated lipoprotein(a) level and therefore is at increased risk for various ASCVD events regardless of his LDL cholesterol or the presence or absence of other risk factors such as elevated body mass index or hypertension.

M. Salama · S. Kumar (✉)
Division of Pediatric Endocrinology, Department of Pediatric and Adolescent Medicine, Mayo Clinic, Rochester, MN, USA
e-mail: salama.mostafa@mayo.edu; kumar.seema@mayo.edu

A. Ashraf, B. Sunil (eds.), *Pediatric Dyslipidemia*,
https://doi.org/10.1007/978-3-031-24113-0_10

Question 2. Of the following, the intervention that has demonstrated maximal lowering of Lp(a) level is:

A. Low fat diet
B. Statins
C. Proprotein convertase subtilisin/kexin type 9 inhibitors
D. Ezetimibe

Answer: C

Critique: Because Lp(a) levels are genetically determined, lifestyle changes including dietary modifications and physical activity don't have significant effect on Lp(a) concentration. Statins and ezetimibe do not lower Lp(a) levels. In contrast, proprotein convertase subtilisin/kexin type 9 (PCSK) inhibitors have been shown to lower Lp(a) levels by 20–30%. However, the contribution of the Lp(a) reduction to their ASCVD risk reduction benefit is unclear at this time, and therefore this class of medications is primarily used with the goal of decreasing LDL cholesterol.

Introduction

Lipoprotein(a) [Lp(a)] was initially identified in 1963 by Kare Berg in immunological experiments of human sera as an antigenic variant of low-density lipoprotein (LDL). He demonstrated that individuals were either Lp(a)+ or Lp(a)- and that there was a higher frequency of Lp(a)+ phenotype in patients with coronary heart disease compared with healthy controls. The Lp(a) gene was subsequently cloned and sequenced in 1987 by Lawn and colleagues. Several observational, Mendelian randomization studies, genome-wide association studies and meta-analyses since then have demonstrated that increased circulating levels of Lp(a) are an independent risk factor for atherosclerotic cardiovascular disease (ASCVD) and valvular aortic stenosis (VAS) [1].

Structure and Metabolism of Lp(a)

Lp(a) has an LDL-like moiety and apo(a) is linked to apo B by a disulfide bond. The LDL-like-moiety has a core of triglycerides and cholesterol esters, surrounded by phospholipids and free cholesterol, and apo B. McLean et al. discovered the structural similarity of Apo(a) with plasminogen which in turn contributes to formation of plasmin, a key to the fibrinolytic cascade. Regions similar to Kringle V and protease regions of plasminogen have also been discovered. There are 10 types of kringle 4-like repeats. The type 2 domain is present in repeated copies varying from 2 to >40.

There is no consensus on whether the LDLR plays a role in the catabolism of Lp(a) as statins that mediate their effect through the LDLR do not alter Lp(a) levels [1, 2].

LPA Gene

In humans, the gene encoding the apo(a) protein, *LPA* was first cloned and sequenced in 1987. The *LPA* gene has up to 70% homology with the human plasminogen gene. The *LPA* gene (MIM 152200; ENSG00000198670) is located in the same cluster as the plasminogen gene, on the long arm of chromosome 6, in the 6q2.6–2.7 region 3 [3]. The *LPA* gene is characterized by 10 different variants present in the KIV domain and by multiple repetitions, ranging from 2 to 43, in the KIV type 2 domain. This gene is inherited as an autosomal codominant trait and there is significant polymorphism. Lp(a) plasma concentrations are highly heritable.

Function of Lp(a)

The exact function of lipoprotein(a) is still unknown. One proposed mechanism underlying the association between elevated levels of Lp(a) and ASCVD risk is the increased procoagulant effect of apo(a) as a result of homology with plasminogen. Additionally, atherogenic and increased proinflammatory effects of the oxidized apolipoprotein B-related phospholipids play an important role. The potential pathophysiologic effects of Lp(a) are summarized in Table 10.1.

Table 10.1 Physiologic effects of Lp(a)

Procoagulant effect of apo A	Proatherogenic effects of Apo B	Proinflammatory effects of apo B
• Decreased plasminogen activation • Decreased fibrinolysis • Enhanced platelet responsiveness and aggregation • Increased endothelial cell plasminogen activator inhibitor −1 expression	• Increased endothelial cell binding • Increased proteoglycan matrix binding • Upregulation of adhesion molecules • Increased necrotic core formation • Enhanced foam cell formation • Increased smooth muscle proliferation • Increased lesion calcification	• Increased oxidized phospholipids • Increased monocyte cytokine release • Increased macrophage interleukin-8 expression • Carrier of monocyte chemoattractant protein 1 • Enhanced chemotaxis of monocytes and transmigration

Adapted from Miksenas, H., J.L. Januzzi, Jr., and P. Natarajan, *Lipoprotein(a) and Cardiovascular Diseases.* JAMA, 2021;326(4): 352–353

Laboratory Measurement of Lipoprotein(a)

Lp(a) is usually measured using antibodies targeting the kringle domains of the apo(a). The measurement of Lp(a) is currently not harmonized or standardized. Several Lp(a) assays are available, and these measure either Lp(a) molar concentration (in nmol/L), Lp(a) mass, and Lp(a) cholesterol. Accurate measurement of Lp(a) is complicated by the heterogeneity of Lp(a) molecular size. Due to the large number of polymorphisms (varying number of kringle domain repeats in the apo[a] protein) in the population, the apo(a) protein can range in size between 240 and 800 kDa, and this heterogeneity can lead to inaccuracies in the measurements. Measurement of Lp(a) using immunoassays calibrated to molar units is recommended to minimize assay inaccuracies caused by apo(a) isoform size. It is recommended that an immunochemical assay calibrated against the World Health Organization/International Federation of Clinical Chemistry and Laboratory Medicine secondary reference material be used and reported in nmol/L. The use of a factor to convert Lp(a) level from mg/dL to nmol/L is discouraged. Lp(a) ≥50 mg/dL or ≥100 nmol/L are suggested as risk factor cut-off points for enhanced ASCVD. This level corresponds to the 80th percentile in populations with predominantly Caucasian individuals. Median Lp(a) is 20 nmol/L in the Caucasian populations. African Americans have approximately threefold higher median Lp(a) levels than Caucasians. However, it is not known if different cut-offs or risk thresholds should be considered for non-Caucasians. Approximately, 20% of individuals have elevated Lp(a) levels (>50 mg/dL or >125 nmol/L). Levels of Lp(a) tend to be stable over time and are transiently affected during inflammatory illness. Fasting is not necessary for measurement of Lp(a).

Association of Lp(a) with Atherosclerotic Cardiovascular Disease

Lp(a) plasma concentrations are thought to be stable from early childhood and therefore high Lp(a) levels represent a lifelong, genetic causal factor for ASCVD, VAS, and mortality [1]. Extremely elevated Lp(a) levels >180 ng/dL (>430 nmol/L) are associated with a lifetime risk of premature ASCVD that is equivalent to that in individuals with heterozygous familial hypercholesterolemia.

Large Mendelian randomization studies and genome-wide association studies demonstrate that high Lp(a) is a causal factor for ASCVD events including myocardial infarction, ischemic stroke, and atherosclerotic stenosis. These also confirm an association between high Lp(a) and aortic valve stenosis, cardiovascular mortality, and all-cause mortality. Genetic variations related to high Lp(a) levels confer the highest risk of ASCVD and VAS among all genetic variations in the human genome.

Meta analyses of population-based studies demonstrate increased risk of ASCVD in patients with Lp(a) above 30 mg/dL (62 nmol/L) and increased risk for ischemic stroke at levels above 50 mg/dL (100 nmol/L). It is important to note that these relationships are independent of the concentrations of other lipids including LDL cholesterol. Large perspective population-based studies demonstrate that individuals with Lp(a) in the top fifth percentile (≥120 mg/dL; 258 nmol/L) had three- to fourfold higher risk of MI and threefold risk for VAS in comparison to those with Lp(a) in the lower 20th percentile (<5 mg/dL; 7 nmol/L). Individuals with highest versus lowest Lp(a) also had 1.6-fold risk of ischemic stroke, 1.5-fold risk of cardiovascular mortality, and 1.24 risk of all-cause mortality.

The distribution of Lp(a) levels differs among ethnic groups with African Americans having higher Lp(a) levels in comparison to Caucasians. However, there is limited evidence for specific cut-off points for high risk based on age, sex, and ethnicity. The 2018 American Heart Association (ACC)/American Heart Association (AHA) Cholesterol Guidelines suggest that Lp(a) values ≥125 nmol/L (or ≥ 50 mg/dL) be considered high risk [4].

Lp(a) in Children

The *LPA* gene is fully expressed by 1–2 years of age and Lp(a) levels reach adult levels by 5 years of age and remain stable throughout the rest of one's life unless there is ongoing inflammation. Elevated levels of the atherogenic Lp(a) start at birth and continue throughout life as the levels are 90% genetically determined with autosomal co-dominant inheritance.

Meta-analyses and case control studies have suggested higher odds of incident idiopathic childhood onset ischemic stroke with high levels of Lp(a) [5]. This increased risk has been attributed to the homology between Lp(a) and plasminogen which inhibits fibrinolysis and increases the risk of thrombosis. However, ASCVD is clinically silent in children with high concentrations of Lp(a). There is need for better data on impact of high Lp(a) on endothelial function during childhood. While one study of flow-mediated dilatation of the brachial artery demonstrated impaired endothelial function in children with familial high Lp(a), another cross-sectional study found no difference in pulse wave velocity or carotid intimal medial thickness between youth with Lp(a) ≥30 mg/dL and those with Lp(a) <30 mg/dL [6].

Interventions for Decreasing Lp(a)

Currently, there is no evidence to demonstrate ASCVD risk reduction as a result of a decrease in the level of Lp(a). The levels of Lp(a) are genetically determined and in general, lifestyle changes including dietary modification and physical activity do not have a significant effect on Lp(a) levels. Statins and ezetimibe do not lower Lp(a) levels. In contrast, proprotein convertase subtilisin/kexin type 9 (PCSK) inhibitors have been shown to lower circulating Lp(a) levels by 20–30%. The contribution of the Lp(a) reduction effect of the PCSK9 inhibitors to their ASCVD risk reduction benefit is unclear currently. Hormone replacement therapy (HRT) in women decreases Lp(a) levels and modifies CVD risk. However, HRT-related adverse events (breast cancer, stroke, thrombosis) outweigh any benefit on CVD and HRT is not recommended for the sole purpose of decreasing Lp(a). Niacin was found to reduce Lp(a) levels by approximately 23% but did not improve ASCVD outcomes and therefore is not recommended. MTP inhibitor, Lomitapide, which is helpful in lowering LDL-C in patients with homozygous familial hypercholesteremia also decreases Lp(a) but is not recommended for ASCVD reduction. Phase II and III trials with mipomersen, an antisense oligonucleotide to apolipoprotein B-100 have shown reduction in Lp(a) levels. CETP inhibitor anacetrapib has also been shown to reduce Lp(a) by up to 40%.

Lipoprotein apheresis can lower circulating Lp(a) levels by 60–75% and is recommended for individuals with elevated Lp(a) who despite maximally tolerated lipid-lowering medications have persistently high LDL cholesterol and history of recurrent ASCVD-related events. Phase 2 clinical trials of apo(a) antisense oligonucleotide have demonstrated reduction of Lp(a) by 35–80%. However further data is necessary before these drugs can be recommended clinically.

Guidelines for Measuring Lp(a) in Adults

There are differences with regard to recommendations by expert groups on measurement of Lp(a) in adults. The European Society of Cardiology and European Atherosclerosis Society guidelines recommend that Lp(a) should be measured universally at least once in each adult's lifetime to detect very high inherited levels of Lp(a) >180 mg/dL (>430 nmol/L) which may pose increased lifetime risk of ASCVD similar to the risk associated with heterozygous familial hypercholesterolemia [7]. Targeted testing is suggested in individuals with a family history of premature CVD, and to reclassify individuals that are borderline between moderate and high-risk category.

In contrast, the National Lipid Association recommends only targeted screening of at-risk adults [1] (Table 10.2).

Table 10.2 National Lipid Association recommendations for Lp(a) screening in adults (age ≥ 20 years)

1. Measurement of Lp(a) is reasonable to refine risk assessment for ASCVD events in adults with – Primary severe hypercholesterolemia (LDL-C ≥ 190 mg/dL) or suspected familial hypercholesterolemia – Family history of first-degree relatives with premature ASCVD – Premature ASCVD (<55 of age in men; <65 years of age in women) – Those at very high risk of ASCVD to better define those who are more likely to benefit from PCSK9 inhibitor therapy
2. Measurement of Lp(a) may be reasonable in cases with. – Family history of elevated Lp(a) – Calcific valvular aortic stenosis – Recurrent or progressive ASCVD, despite optimal lipid-lowering therapy – Less than anticipated LDL cholesterol-lowering despite good adherence to LDL cholesterol-lowering therapy – Borderline (5–7.4%) or intermediate (7.5–19.9%) 19 years. ASCVD risk when the decision to use a statin is uncertain.

Adapted from Wilson, D.P., et al., Use of Lipoprotein(a) in clinical practice: A biomarker whose time has come. A scientific statement from the National Lipid Association. J Clin Lipidol, 2019;13(3): 374–392

Guidelines for Measuring Lp(a) in Youth

The 2019 American Heart Association scientific statement for cardiovascular risk reduction in high-risk pediatric patients noted that elevated Lp(a) "could represent a useful marker to identify young familial hypercholesterolemia patients at very high risk of premature CVD" [8]. Although, the 2011 National Heart, Lung, and Blood Institute Expert Panel emphasized the importance of global risk assessment and early intervention in youth with moderate-to-high risk medical conditions such as diabetes mellitus and diseases associated with chronic inflammation, such as systemic lupus erythematosus, measurement of Lp(a) was only suggested in children who had experienced either hemorrhagic or ischemic stroke [9]. Reasons to not recommend universal Lp(a) screening in youth include the absence of targeted treatment to lower Lp(a) levels, creating fear and overtreatment of young children found to have elevated levels and the absence of well-defined risk thresholds and population norms in children. The National Lipid Association suggests targeted screening in youth (age <20 years) (Table 10.3). Other experts however have recommended that Lp(a) measurement also be considered in patients with moderate to high risk factors and risk conditions [10] (Table 10.3).

The recommended approach to ASCVD reduction in patients with high Lp(a) is to improve modifiable risk factors such as excessive weight, unhealthy diet, sedentary lifestyle, and elevated blood pressure and aim at aggressive lowering of LDL cholesterol as per the 2019 American Heart Association Guidelines.

Table 10.3 Recommendations for Lp(a) screening in youth <20 years of age

Measurement of Lp(a) may be reasonable in youth with	
1	Clinically suspected or genetically confirmed FH
2	Family history of first-degree relatives with premature ASCVD (<55 years of age in men, <65 years of age in women)
3	An unknown cause of ischemic stroke
4	A parent or sibling found to have an elevated Lp(a)
5	All patients with moderate to high risk factors or risk conditions
Moderate risk conditions or factors	
–	Hypertension not requiring drug treatment
–	High-density lipoprotein cholesterol <40 mg/dL
–	BMI ≥95th percentile to <97th percentile
–	Nephrotic syndrome
–	Chronic inflammatory condition (systemic lupus erythematosus, juvenile rheumatoid arthritis
–	Kawasaki disease with regressed coronary aneurysms
–	HIV infection
High-risk conditions or factors	
–	Hypertension requiring medical treatment
–	Active smoking
–	BMI ≥ 97th percentile
–	Diabetes mellitus
–	Chronic renal disease/end stage kidney disease/post-kidney transplant
–	Ischemic stroke of unknown origin
–	Kawasaki disease with coronary aneurysms
–	Post-orthotopic heart transplant

Adapted from Kohn, B., A.P. Ashraf, and D.P. Wilson, *Should Lipoprotein(a) be Measured in Youth?* J Pediatr, 2021;228:285–289

Future Directions

Although Lp(a) has been shown to be an independent risk factor for ASCVD, additional evidence is needed regarding the cost–benefit ratio of early testing and effect of Lp(a) reduction on ASCVD outcomes. Additionally, there is need for larger studies to determine if the Lp(a) cut-offs for increased ASCVD risk vary with ethnicity.

Summary

- Lipoprotein(a) is a spherical macromolecular complex with a structure similar to that of low-density lipoproteins that is synthesized in the liver and secreted with different isoform sizes.
- Isoform size variations exist within populations.
- Lipoprotein (a) consists of apolipoprotein(a) which is covalently bound by a single disulfide bond to apo B. Apo(a) contains 10 different types of kringle 4-like repeats (not V). There are also regions homologous to the kringle 5 and protease regions of plasminogen.

- The measurement of Lp(a) is not standardized and immunoassays have the potential for bias due to the presence of variable numbers of repeated units in differently sized apo(a) isoforms. Measurement of Lp(a) using immunoassays calibrated to molar units is recommended to minimize assay inaccuracies caused by apo(a) isoform size.
- LPA gene is located on the long arm of chromosome 6. This gene is inherited as an autosomal codominant trait with significant polymorphism. Gene expression starts by 1–2 years of age and adult levels are attained by 5 years of age.
- Lp(a) is an independent risk factor for ASCVD events including myocardial infarction and valvular aortic stenosis in adults regardless of LDL-C level. There is also strong evidence linking higher levels of Lp(a) with the development of ischemic strokes during childhood.
- The unique structure of Lp(a) plays an important role in mediating fibrinolytic system inhibition, increasing platelet activation and adhesion molecules on the endothelial surface and vascular smooth muscle proliferation. These effects are the underlying mechanisms for the development of atherosclerotic cardiovascular disease (ASCVD).
- The distribution of Lp(a) levels differs among ethnic groups with African Americans having higher median Lp(a) levels relative to Caucasians. There is limited evidence on specific cut points for high risk based on demographic variables. Most studies suggest a single cut-off for Lp(a) between100 and 125 nmol/L (or ≥50 mg/dL) for high ASCVD risk in all ethnic groups.
- Because Lp(a) levels are mainly genetically determined, lifestyle changes including dietary changes and physical activity do not have a significant effect on Lp(a) concentration. Statins and ezetimibe also do not reduce Lp(a) levels. PCSK9 inhibitors have been shown to decrease Lp(a) levels by 20–30%.
- Currently, there is no data to demonstrate reduction in ASCVD outcomes as a result of a decrease in the level of Lp(a) independent of the effect of the treatment on other lipoproteins including LDL cholesterol.
- The current guidelines state that Lp(a) screening "may be reasonable" for pediatric patients from 2 to 20 years of age with clinically suspected or genetically confirmed familial hypercholesterolemia, family history of first degree relative with premature ASCVD, unknown cause of ischemic stroke or a family history of elevated Lp(a) level in parent or sibling.
- Guidelines with regard to screening for elevated Lp(a) in adults vary with some experts suggesting universal screening at least once in each adult's lifetime and others suggesting targeted screening in selected patients including those with primary severe hypercholesterolemia or suspected FH, premature ASCVD in the absence of additional risk factors and family history of a first-degree relative with premature ACVD.
- The recommended approach to ASCVD reduction in patients with high Lp(a) is to improve modifiable risk factors such as excessive weight, unhealthy diet, sedentary lifestyle, and elevated blood pressure and aim at aggressive lowering of LDL cholesterol as according to the 2019 American Heart Association Guidelines.

References

1. Wilson DP, et al. Use of lipoprotein(a) in clinical practice: a biomarker whose time has come. A scientific statement from the National Lipid Association. J Clin Lipidol. 2019;13(3):374–92.
2. Jang AY, et al. Lipoprotein(a) and cardiovascular diseases-revisited. Circ J. 2020;84(6):867–74.
3. Schmidt K, et al. Structure, function, and genetics of lipoprotein (a). J Lipid Res. 2016;57(8):1339–59.
4. Grundy SM, et al. 2018 AHA/ACC/AACVPR/AAPA/ABC/ACPM/ADA/AGS/APhA/ASPC/NLA/PCNA guideline on the Management of Blood Cholesterol: a report of the American College of Cardiology/American Heart Association task force on clinical practice guidelines. Circulation. 2019;139(25):e1082–143.
5. Nowak-Göttl U, et al. Lipoprotein (a) and genetic polymorphisms of clotting factor V, prothrombin, and methylenetetrahydrofolate reductase are risk factors of spontaneous ischemic stroke in childhood. Blood. 1999;94(11):3678–82.
6. Qayum O, et al. Lipoprotein (a): examination of cardiovascular risk in a pediatric referral population. Pediatr Cardiol. 2018;39(8):1540–6.
7. Mach F, et al. 2019 ESC/EAS guidelines for the management of dyslipidaemias: lipid modification to reduce cardiovascular risk. Eur Heart J. 2020;41(1):111–88.
8. de Ferranti SD, et al. Cardiovascular risk reduction in high-risk pediatric patients: a scientific statement from the American Heart Association. Circulation. 2019;139(13):e603–34.
9. Expert Panel on Integrated Guidelines for Cardiovascular, et al. Expert panel on integrated guidelines for cardiovascular health and risk reduction in children and adolescents: summary report. Pediatrics. 2011;128(Suppl 5):S213–56.
10. Kohn B, Ashraf AP, Wilson DP. Should lipoprotein(a) be measured in youth? J Pediatr. 2021;228:285–9.

Chapter 11
Rare Genetic Dyslipidemia

Christy Foster, Bhuvana Sunil, and Ambika Ashraf

Introduction

Common lipid disorders have been extensively discussed in previous chapters. The focus of this chapter is to describe clinically relevant rare genetic dyslipidemias.

Sitosterolemia

Sitosterolemia is characterized by significant elevations in plant sterols (beta-sitosterol, campesterol, and stigmasterol). This should be suspected when patients are not responding with cholestrol lowering to statin therapy or when demonstrates a remarkably excellent response to dietary modifications or to ezetimibe. Affected patients absorb plant sterols excessively without restriction. Often asymptomatic clinically, these disorders can present with tendon or tuberous xanthomas and premature atherosclerosis [1]. Other clinical findings may include joint stiffness, hemolytic anemia with stomatocytosis, macrothrombocytopenia, and splenomegaly [1]. There is significant phenotypic heterogeneity. Laboratory evaluations may show elevated low-density lipoprotein cholesterol (LDL-C) and total cholesterol.

This autosomal recessive condition is caused by biallelic pathogenic variants in *ABCG5* or *ABCG8* encoding the intestinal and hepatic heterodimer ABCG5

C. Foster · A. Ashraf (✉)
University of Alabama at Birmingham, Birmingham, AL, USA
e-mail: cafoster@uabmc.edu; aashraf@uabmc.edu

B. Sunil
Mary Bridge Children's Hospital, Tacoma, WA, USA
e-mail: Bhuvana.sunil@multicare.org

A. Ashraf, B. Sunil (eds.), *Pediatric Dyslipidemia*,
https://doi.org/10.1007/978-3-031-24113-0_11

(sterolin 1)/ABCG8 (sterolin 2) efflux transporters [1]. Dietary sterols normally passively enter the intestinal cells and are then eliminated out into the gut lumen by the ATP-binding cassette (ABC) transporter proteins. In sitosterolemia, impaired ABC transporter protein causes increased intestinal absorption of sitosterols and decreased biliary excretion, leading to elevated plasma levels of plant sterols and stanols in plasma and tissues [2].

These patients often do not respond to statin therapy. Their lipid abnormalities responds to a diet that is low in plant sterols. Avoiding or reducing shellfish and plant sterols, i.e., vegetable oils, margarine, nuts, seeds, avocados, and chocolate is recommended. Treatment with sterol absorption inhibitor ezetimibe is effective. Bile acid sequestrants such as cholestyramine (8–15 g/day) can be tried. Monitoring can be done with measurement of plant sterols levels [1].

Lipodystrophy

Lipodystrophy syndromes are heterogeneous disorders characterized by deficiency of adipose tissue without evidence of nutritional deprivation or a catabolic state. These conditions can lead to metabolic complications such as insulin resistance and hypertriglyceridemia. Loss of adipose tissue results in a decrease of leptin (hypoleptinemia). The lack of adipose tissue results in storage of triglycerides in liver and skeletal muscle and pancreas leading to insulin resistance, hypertriglyceridemia, and hepatic steatosis [3].

There are four major subtypes, namely congenital generalized lipodystrophy, acquired generalized lipodystrophy, familial partial lipodystrophy, and acquired partial lipodystrophy. Generalized lipodystrophy should be suspected when a patient demonstrates near total lack of subcutaneous adipose tissue, prominent muscles, accelerated growth, voracious appetite, acanthosis, and acromegaloid appearance. Associated comorbidities include diabetes mellitus, severe hypertriglyceridemia, non-alcoholic steatohepatitis, or polycystic ovary syndrome [4].

Congenital lipodystrophy is a rare autosomal recessive disorder associated with near total absence of adipose tissue. Common types are type 1 is due to *AGPAT-2* and type 2 is due to *BSCL2* mutations. Progeroid syndrome is associated with features including short stature, alopecia, sclerodermatous skin changes, osteoporosis, and joint contractures. Metabolic syndrome is usually not associated [3].

Compared with congenital generalized lipodystrophy, acquired generalized lipodystrophy has a later onset with the loss of adipose tissue occurring in childhood or adolescence. Frequently associated comorbidities include insulin resistance, hypertriglyceridemia, and hepatic steatosis. It is more common in women than men [4]. Acquired generalized lipodystrophy (AGL) can be secondary to autoimmune disease due to activation of the complement pathway. The three subtypes of AGL include panniculitis, autoimmune, and idiopathic [3].

Familial partial lipodystrophy encompasses a number of conditions sharing a cushingoid appearance, i.e., dorso cervical fat pad and obesity. The loss of adipose tissue occurs in childhood and adolescence and is associated with excess fat in the neck, face, and in the abdomen. There are eight subtypes of familial partial lipodystrophy. The classic phenotype associated with type 2 familial partial lipodystrophy (Dunnigan type) is attributed to variants in exon 8 of the *LMNA* gene. The phenotype may include defined musculature, hypertrophy of calves, and valvular heart disease. In type 3 familial partial lipodystrophy, the loss of adipose tissue occurs in adulthood. Cardiometabolic complications are severe. Type 4 lipodystrophy will show severe dyslipidemia and insulin resistance [3].

The diagnosis of lipodystrophy is suspected based on the history, physical examination, and features of metabolic syndrome. When suspected, a thorough pedigree analysis and genetic testing can help make the diagnosis.

Currently, treatment for lipodystrophy is focused on lifestyle changes. Recombinant leptin (metreleptin) is approved by the Food and Drug Administration in 2014 to treat the metabolic complications of leptin deficiency in patients with generalized lipodystrophy (congenital or acquired generalized lipodystrophy, non-HIV-related). It is not approved for the partial lipodystrophy yet, clinical trials are ongoing [5]. Leptin treatment has been associated with lower hemoglobin A1c, fasting glucose, and triglycerides, and improved liver volume [3].

Hypoalphalipoproteinemia

High-density lipoprotein (HDL) is a spherical lipoprotein which contains ~20% cholesterol. The major proteins of HDL are apo A-I and apo A-II.

Familial HDL deficiency is typically secondary to mutations in *ABCA1* or the *APOA1* gene. These mutations are typically inherited in an autosomal dominant pattern [6]. Heterozygotes can have ~30% lower HDL-C levels.

Laboratory studies include a low measured HDL-C, i.e., ≤25 mg/dL [6]. Often patients will have normal triglycerides (TG) and LDL-C. Affected patients may develop cardiovascular disease often before the age of 50. In 1982, Norum et al. described two sisters with marked HDL deficiency, planar xanthomas, and premature CVD. The siblings were found to have undetectable plasma apoA-I and apoC-III. The patients required bypass surgery at ages 29 and 30 years [6]. Patients with familial HDL deficiency should have their LDL-C levels optimized with statin therapy, and if necessary, with other agents. Genetic counseling should include discussion of the risk of affected offspring being 50%.

Tangier Disease

Tangier disease (TD) is an autosomal recessive disease where there is significant accumulation of cholesterol esters and low HDL-C [6]. This condition was first described by Fredrickson et al. in 1961 in two siblings with enlarged tonsils with yellow-orange discoloration and hepatomegaly. Peripheral neuropathies including a syringomyelia-like neuropathy (SMLN) and distal symmetric polyneuropathies can be seen [6]. Clinical manifestations include orange tonsils, premature ASCVD risk, syringomyelia like neuropathy, corneal clouding, hepatosplenomegaly, and increased risk of diabetes, thrombocytopenia, and anemia.

TD is associated with a mutation in the gene encoding ATP-cassette binding transporter 1 (*ABCA 1*). *ABCA1* is the first step of the reverse cholesterol transport and is important in the intake of cholesterol and phospholipid to the lipoprotein receptors (particularly apo-A1). Hence free cholesterol cannot be transported out of the cell. The impaired interaction between *ABCA1* and apoA-I is believed to result in the accumulation of cholesterol esters and thus foam-cell formation [6].

Management and close follow-up of the manifestations include tonsillectomy in those with airway obstruction, bracing and exercise to improve the peripheral neuropathy, and corneal transplants for corneal opacities. For their lipid dysfunction, statin therapy and a low-fat diet are recommended [7]. Genetic counseling is also recommended as each sibling of an affected patient has a 25% chance of being affected. They also have a 50% chance of being a carrier, leading to HDL levels which are ~50% of normal [7].

LCAT Deficiency

LCAT deficiency is another rare genetic dyslipidemia. This can occur either in the complete form, which is associated with multiple systemic morbidities including anemia and renal failure, whereas partial LCAT deficiency has a milder presentation with corneal opacities, hence named as "Fisheye Disease" (FED).

FED was first described in a male Norwegian patient and his three daughters. Signs will often begin to develop in early adolescence. Laboratory findings show normal serum cholesterol, elevated TG, elevated VLDL, elevated LDL-C, and significant HDL-C deficiency (HDL <10 mg/dL) [8]. These patients can be at risk for premature cardiovascular disease and renal disease.

Alpha-LCAT is an enzyme responsible for attaching cholesterol esterification and promotes the formation of HDL-C. With this enzyme deficiency, unesterified free cholesterol is deposited in the corneal stroma, kidneys, and erythrocytes, because patients with FED cannot esterify free cholesterol contained in HDL particles [9]. This condition is inherited in an autosomal recessive pattern.

Treatment may require corneal transplant given the severe opacification which can occur. Renal transplant may also need to be considered in severe cases. Lipid-lowering medications are critical in the management of these patients.

Apolipoprotein A-I Deficiency

In 1982, hypoapolipoprotein A-I was described where a female patient was found to have significantly low HDL-C and low TG levels. The increased ratio of total cholesterol (TC) to HDL-C predisposes these patients to cardiovascular disease. Clinical findings would include corneal arcus, plantar xanthomas, severe diffuse coronary disease, and peripheral atherosclerosis [6]. Less commonly, this condition can lead to neurosensory impairment such as hearing loss, retinopathy, or cerebellar ataxia [6].

Laboratory findings will show a plasma apoA-I level will be undetectable. Triglycerides will be low while there will be normal LDL-C. The disease is secondary to mutations in the *APOA1* gene. This condition is inherited in an autosomal dominant pattern. ApoA-1 promotes the movement of cholesterol and phospholipids from the inside to outer surface of the cell. It is a cofactor for lecithin cholesterol acyltransferase. These cholesterol and phospholipid substrate will then undergo cholesterol esterification to be integrated into HDL-C [10].

Several medications can be utilized to improve the cardiovascular risk. Statins can be utilized to lower the total cholesterol and will be the most effective way to lower the ratio of TC:HDL-C. Niacin can be used to increase the HDL-C.

Abeta and Hypobetalipoproteinemia

Low LDL cholesterol results from familial abetalipoproteinemia or hypobetalipoproteinemia. Hypobetalipoproteinemia is due to an abnormality in apoB leading to very low levels of apoB containing lipoproteins. This disorder is associated with longevity and does not cause any longterm adverse outcomes.

Familial Abetalipoproteinemia is due to abnormal assembly of VLDL due to a defect in MTP (mitochondrial triglyceride transport protein). This condition was first reported in the medical literature in 1950 by Bassen and Kornzweig. Clinical symptoms can include gastrointestinal disease due to poor fat malabsorption such as foul-smelling stools, diarrhea, and abdominal distension [11]. Neurological complications can occur that resemble spinocerebellar degeneration. Skeletal abnormalities including lordosis, kyphoscoliosis, or clubfoot. Some individuals could include retinitis pigmentosa due to vitamin A and E deficiency. These patients can also develop acanthocytosis (burr-shaped red blood cells).

The phenotype is characterized by low triglycerides, extremely low total cholesterol, absent plasma VLDL, LDL, and apoB. Abetalipoproteinemia is caused by mutations in the *MTTP* gene and is inherited in an autosomal recessive pattern [11]. Mutations in the gene will lead to low levels of functional MTP which will hinder the liver and intestines from making apoB containing lipoproteins including VLDL, LDL, and chylomicrons.

Treatment at this time is focused on supportive care for the symptoms that develop. This includes seeing subspecialists such as lipidologists, hepatologists for liver disease, ophthalmologists, and neurologists. Most affected individuals respond to a diet low in fat, especially long-chain saturated fatty acids. Diets in infancy may need supplementation with medium-chain fatty acids to promote normal growth and development. Supplementation with fat-soluble vitamins may also be indicated [12].

Cerebro-Tendinous Xanthomatosis

Cerebro-tendinous xanthomatosis (CTX) is an autosomal recessive genetic disorder. Patients will develop neurological symptoms including loss of cognitive skills, coordination of balance. Mental dysfunction can start in puberty [13]. Psychiatric symptoms such as depression, aggression, and dementia can develop over time if left untreated. Early in childhood, cataracts may appear. Benign fatty tumors (xanthomas) will often develop at the ends of tendons in the second and third decade of life. Cholestatic liver disease develops early due to the impairment of bile salt being released by the liver, leading to hepatosplenomegaly. Cardiovascular disease is also possible due to intimal thickening of the arteries.

This disorder is caused by an abnormality in the *CYP27A1* gene. This variation will lead to a deficiency of the mitochondrial enzyme 27-hydroxylase [13]. This deficiency will prevent cholesterol from conversion into a bile acid called chenodeoxycholic acid [14]. The deposit will then accumulate in the nerve cells leading to damage to the nervous system, tendons, lens of the eye, and arteries [15]. CTX can lead to neurological pathology including seizures, ataxia, and cognitive impairment. Due to the biochemical defect, the cholestanol concentration in plasma is high, while the plasma cholesterol concentration is normal to low [15].

Therapy currently concentrates on oral bile acid replacement therapy. Early identification and initiation of treatment is critical for disease complication prevention. In 2009, the FDA approved a synthetic form of chenodeoxycholic acid (Chenodal) which is typically used first line for patients with CTX [12]. Statin therapy could lead to the increased LDL receptor activity which could increase cholesterol uptake and worsen CTX. Cholic acid, another bile acid, has been used to treat pediatric patients with CTX [15].

Lipoprotein X

Lipoprotein X is a lipoprotein anomaly which will lead to an increase in cholesterol. LpX is a phospholipid and free cholesterol sphere with a hollow core. Typically, LpX is seen in biliary obstruction when the liver is still healthy enough to synthesize bile constituents of bile acids, free cholesterol, and phospholipids that then reflux into the plasma. In this condition, lipid factions from the bile salts will spill into the plasma and bind to albumin to create LpX. The lipid composition of LpX comprises approximately equal parts (40–45% each) of free cholesterol and phospholipids, less than 5% cholesterol esters and negligible amounts of triglycerides [15]. Patients with this condition are at risk for hyperviscosity syndrome due to the elevated cholesterol including pulmonary embolism.

Lipoprotein X is a lamellar vesicle with approximately equal amounts of free cholesterol and phospholipids. This molecule involves a lack of apolipoprotein B (apoB). The absence of apoB means that the lipoprotein cannot bind to hepatic molecules, Lipoprotein X can only be removed by plasmapheresis [16].

Pharmacotherapy that is generally used in hypercholesterolemia such as statin therapy are ineffective in treating this condition as lipoprotein X does not have any apoB and thus the statins will not affect the removal of this lipoprotein by the liver. Ezetimibe is not as effective either as it will target the dietary absorption of cholesterol which plays a minimal role in the conformation of lipoprotein X. Fibrates can be considered as they have an anti-cholestatic and anti-inflammatory effect in liver disease [16].

Clinical Case

A previously healthy 13-year-old girl presented for evaluation of dyslipidemia. The patient reports gradual loss of her body fat and athletic appearance even though not exercising regularly. Family history is unremarkable. On physical examination, her blood pressure and growth parameters are normal. Her current BMI is at the 95th percentile for age. On exam, she acanthosis nigricans, acne, fullness to her face and neck, and muscular upper and lower extremities. She has a HbA1C of 6.1%, ALT of 195 U/L and AST of 124 U/L.

Her lipid profile result is below:

Total cholesterol: 240 mg/dL

Triglycerides: 350 mg/dL

LDL-C: 127 mg/dL

HDL-C: 43 mg/dL

Non-HDL-C: 197 mg/dL

Questions to consider:

- *What is the patient's likely diagnosis?*
- *What further testing might be indicated by this patient?*

Answer: The patient likely has familial partial lipodystrophy. This condition has been inherited most often in an autosomal dominant pattern, that presents with gradual loss of adipose tissue around puberty. These patients often are at risk for metabolic syndrome including insulin resistance. It is important to rule out acquired lipodystrophy.

Screening for associated comorbidities such as non alcoholic fatty liver disease, insulin resistance, and type 2 diabetes are important.

Conclusions

- Genetic etiology should be considered in the setting of dyslipidemia.
- Distinct phenotypic features may be present in some of the rare genetic dyslipidemias.

References

1. Myrie SB, Steiner RD, Mymin D. Sitosterolemia. In: Adam MP, et al., editors. GeneReviews((R)). Seattle: University of Washington; 1993.
2. Park JH, et al. Sitosterolemia presenting with severe hypercholesterolemia and intertriginous xanthomas in a breastfed infant: case report and brief review. J Clin Endocrinol Metab. 2014;99(5):1512–8.
3. Brown RJ, et al. The diagnosis and Management of Lipodystrophy Syndromes: a multi-society practice guideline. J Clin Endocrinol Metab. 2016;101(12):4500–11.
4. Araujo-Vilar D, Santini F. Diagnosis and treatment of lipodystrophy: a step-by-step approach. J Endocrinol Investig. 2019;42(1):61–73.
5. Brown RJ, et al. Effects of Metreleptin in pediatric patients with lipodystrophy. J Clin Endocrinol Metab. 2017;102(5):1511–9.
6. Mercan M, et al. Peripheral neuropathy in Tangier disease: a literature review and assessment. J Peripher Nerv Syst. 2018;23(2):88–98.
7. Burnett JR, et al. Tangier disease. In: Adam MP, et al., editors. GeneReviews((R)). Seattle: University of Washington; 1993.
8. Kanai M, et al. Clinical features and visual function in a patient with fish-eye disease: quantitative measurements and optical coherence tomography. Am J Ophthalmol Case Rep. 2018;10:137–41.
9. Rousset X, et al. Lecithin: cholesterol acyltransferase--from biochemistry to role in cardiovascular disease. Curr Opin Endocrinol Diabetes Obes. 2009;16(2):163–71.
10. Yui Y, et al. Serum prostacyclin stabilizing factor is identical to apolipoprotein A-I (Apo A-I). A novel function of Apo A-I. J Clin Invest. 1988;82(3):803–7.
11. Welty FK. Hypobetalipoproteinemia and abetalipoproteinemia. Curr Opin Lipidol. 2014;25(3):161–8.
12. Lee J, Hegele RA. Abetalipoproteinemia and homozygous hypobetalipoproteinemia: a framework for diagnosis and management. J Inherit Metab Dis. 2014;37(3):333–9.
13. Carson BE, De Jesus O. Cerebrotendinous Xanthomatosis. Treasure Island (FL): StatPearls; 2021.
14. Bjorkhem I. Cerebrotendinous xanthomatosis. Curr Opin Lipidol. 2013;24(4):283–7.
15. Nie S, et al. Cerebrotendinous xanthomatosis: a comprehensive review of pathogenesis, clinical manifestations, diagnosis, and management. Orphanet J Rare Dis. 2014;9:179.
16. Kattah L, et al. Hypercholesterolemia due to lipoprotein X: case report and thematic review. Clin Med Insights Endocrinol Diabetes. 2019;12:1179551419878687.

Index

A. Ashraf, B. Sunil (eds.), *Pediatric Dyslipidemia*,
https://doi.org/10.1007/978-3-031-24113-0

GPSR Compliance

The European Union's (EU) General Product Safety Regulation (GPSR) is a set of rules that requires consumer products to be safe and our obligations to ensure this.

If you have any concerns about our products, you can contact us on ProductSafety@springernature.com

In case Publisher is established outside the EU, the EU authorized representative is:

Springer Nature Customer Service Center GmbH
Europaplatz 3
69115 Heidelberg, Germany

Batch number: 10732090

Printed by Printforce, the Netherlands